From the Editors of **Hea**

D0069959

The Carb Lovers DIET

POCKET GUIDE

THE QUICK & EASY WAY TO LOSE 15•35•100+ LBS AND NEVER FEEL HUNGRY!

By **Ellen Kunes,** *Editor in Chief,*
and **Frances Largeman-Roth, RD,**
Health *magazine*

OXMOOR HOUSE

ISBN-13: 978-0-8487-3527-2
ISBN-10: 0-8487-3527-7
Library of Congress Control Number: 2010940722
Printed in the United States of America
First printing 2011

This book is intended as a general reference
only, and is not to be used as a substitute for medical advice
or treatment. We urge you to consult your physician
regarding any individual medical conditions or specific
health-related issues or questions.

Contents

Yes, You Can Lose Weight Eating Carbs!
(And Keep It Off, Too!)

By Ellen Kunes, Editor in Chief, HEALTH magazine
Editorial Director, Health.com

READ THIS IF YOU'RE CARBO-PHOBIC! If you're like me, you've spent years avoiding all of your favorite carb-filled foods—delicious, filling pastas, yummy pizzas, hamburgers with their buns on, sandwiches with chips on the side.

It's not surprising: We've been told for more than two decades that these scrumptious basics of a happy, pleasure-filled life will pile on the pounds. **But here's the big news:** Groundbreaking research reveals that our beloved, carb-filled foods will *not* make us fat. Instead, they can actually make us *thin*.

CarbLovers Tip

Want even *more* grab-and-go, restaurant, and grocery items to choose from? Log on to carblovers.com for a free guide!

All these new studies are cited at **carblovers.com,** but here's the bottom line: The best and brightest minds in nutrition science today agree that carbs can shrink fat cells (especially around your belly), help burn more fat, and keep you feeling full longer than other foods.

But all the studies in the world wouldn't have made *The CarbLovers Diet* a success if we didn't include a proven diet plan—one with delicious, easy meals that you can enjoy for the rest of your life.

Many of you were such big *CarbLovers* fans that you told us you wanted more diet menus, more recipes, more grab-and-go options. So that's what you'll love about *The CarbLovers Diet Pocket Guide.*

With its new breakthrough weight-loss plan, quick and tasty recipes, complete shopping guides, and expanded list of *CarbLovers*-approved grocery and restaurant foods, *The CarbLovers Diet Pocket Guide* will make it even easier for you to enjoy *CarbLovers* on the go. We've included recipes you're going to want to make right this minute (like our delicious Steel-Cut Oatmeal with Salted Caramel Topping for breakfast, the ultimate CarbLovers Club Sandwich for lunch, and my favorite, the Sausage, Tomato, White Bean & Corkscrew Pasta Toss, for dinner). I know you'll love these additions as much as I do!

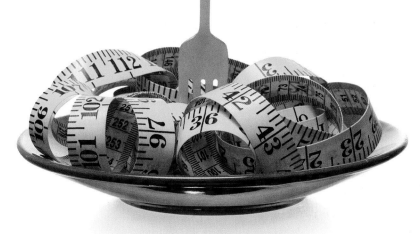

Ready, Set, Eat Potato Chips With The Pocket Guide!

MANY OF YOU HAVE ALREADY TRIED (AND DROPPED POUNDS ON) *The CarbLovers Diet.* Congrats! This guide will make it easier to keep eating what you love and maintain your weight (or lose even more).

If you're getting ready to start *CarbLovers* for the first time, it may take a few days for you to adjust to a new reality: that **carbs are the best things that ever happened to your waistline.** You'll enjoy delicious foods and—this is key—up the percentage of a type of carb called Resistant Starch in your diet. Resistant Starch is getting lots of press these days, because it's a boon for weight loss (and your overall health). It doesn't get absorbed into the bloodstream in the small intestine, like other foods—but it does shrink fat cells, preserve muscle, stoke your metabolism, and make you feel full longer. Best of all, foods filled with Resistant Starch aren't fancy or expensive! They're breads, pasta, cereals, potatoes, even potato chips—foods you already have at home or can easily pick up at the supermarket.

The CarbLovers Diet Pocket Guide Diet Plan has two parts, and both come with a shopping list, a meal plan that offers recipes and grab-and-go options (for those days when you don't want to cook), and nutrition information about what you're eating, including the amount of Resistant Starch when available.

The *CarbLovers Diet* begins with a 7-Day *CarbLovers* Kickstart Plan. The one we created for this guide will help you quickly knock off up to 6 pounds and reduce belly bloat, all while feeling satisfied.

After you've tasted success on the 7-Day *CarbLovers* Kickstart Plan, you're ready for the life-changing 21-Day *CarbLovers* Immersion Plan. The version created for *The CarbLovers Diet Pocket Guide* will ease you back into "normal eating" with delicious, portion-controlled recipes and grocery options. By the end of these three weeks, you'll have lost up to another 6 pounds!

5 Rules of The CarbLovers Diet

Rule 1: Eat a CarbStar at every meal. Resistant Starch carbs are the weight-busting champs of this diet. These "CarbStars" include bananas, oatmeal, beans and lentils, potatoes, whole-grain pasta, barley, brown rice, peas, rye and pumpernickel bread, polenta, and potato chips (yes, you read that right—potato chips!).

Rule 2: Balance your plate. CarbStars should take up about a quarter of your plate. The rest will be filled with tasty weight-loss boosters such as lean meats, fruit, veggies, and low-fat dairy products.

Rule 3: Be smart about portions. Yes, you can eat carbs, but stick with the portions our experts dish out. Trust us: You won't feel hungry!

Rule 4: Never deprive yourself. On *CarbLovers,* you can have dessert, wine, even chocolate. That's because the more we restrict "forbidden" foods, the more likely we are to binge on them.

Rule 5: Stock up. Some yummy foods appear frequently on this diet. Use our shopping guides to shop smarter.

CarbLovers Tip

If you're on a budget, try buying your dry goods—pasta, oats, brown rice—in bulk. Then store them in airtight containers away from heat and light. This helps them last much longer. Label each container with the name of the food, the correct serving size, and cooking instructions.

What's on the CarbLovers Menu?

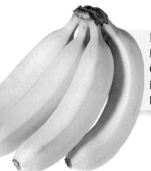

Fruit! Certain types of fruit, especially bananas, are rich in Resistant Starch. Others pack pectin, a type of fiber found in the rinds and skins of fruit that may block fat storage.

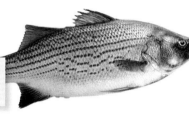

Fish! Cold-water fish contain omega-3 fatty acids, which switch on enzymes that trigger fat-burning in cells.

Beans! These foods contain fat-busting fiber. One study found that every 1-gram increase in fiber consumed correlated with a half-pound of weight loss!

Meat and dairy! Both contain conjugated linoleic acid, a fat that is thought to help blood glucose enter body cells so it can be burned for energy and not stored as fat.

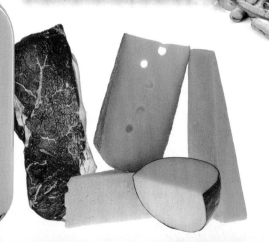

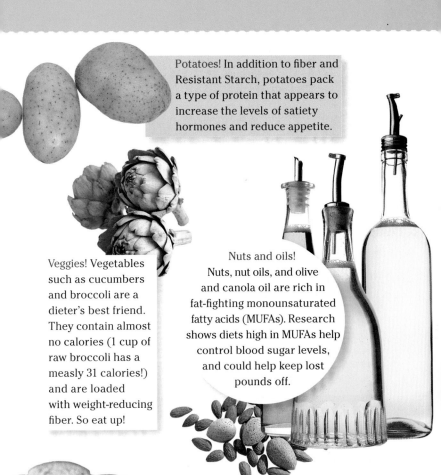

Potatoes! In addition to fiber and Resistant Starch, potatoes pack a type of protein that appears to increase the levels of satiety hormones and reduce appetite.

Veggies! Vegetables such as cucumbers and broccoli are a dieter's best friend. They contain almost no calories (1 cup of raw broccoli has a measly 31 calories!) and are loaded with weight-reducing fiber. So eat up!

Nuts and oils! Nuts, nut oils, and olive and canola oil are rich in fat-fighting monounsaturated fatty acids (MUFAs). Research shows diets high in MUFAs help control blood sugar levels, and could help keep lost pounds off.

Bread, rice, pasta, and whole grains! *The CarbLovers Diet* celebrates tortillas, bread, and pasta—especially the whole-grain kinds rich in Resistant Starch and fiber. Research shows that people who consume more whole grains tend to weigh less than people who skip them.

The Resistant Starch Secret: Blast Fat, Feel Happy!

YOU'VE PROBABLY HEARD THE TERM "RESISTANT STARCH," the power player in *The CarbLovers Diet*. Resistant Starch has generated lots of interest for a very good reason!

This amazing fat-burning carb can be found in many of your favorite foods (see Top Resistant Starch Foods, page 14). And it isn't hard to get enough Resistant Starch to feel fuller and see dramatic weight-loss results.

CarbLovers Tip

What's the fastest way to make sure you're getting enough Resistant Starch? Eat one slightly green banana a day, either in a Banana Shake (page 57) or as a snack. That will guarantee you 12.5 grams of Resistant Starch—all you need that day!

Resistant Starch isn't new or some trendy diet gimmick. It has been the subject of nearly 200 respected studies at top medical centers around the world. Research shows Resistant Starch is a weight-loss powerhouse, primarily because it does not get absorbed into the bloodstream or broken down into glucose. Therefore, it does not raise blood sugar. It travels through your digestive system nearly intact, triggering incredible weight-loss benefits.

Resistant Starch helps you get slim—and stay slim—by:
■ Turning on enzymes that melt fat, especially in the belly area
■ Encouraging your liver to switch to a fat-burning state
■ Boosting satiety hormones, which make you feel full longer

How Much Resistant Starch Do You Need to Eat?

Probably more than you're eating now—and that's good news. The *CarbLovers* menu includes 10 to 15 grams each day of Resistant Starch, served up in delicious recipes like Chicken Pasta Primavera (page 93) and Coconut French Toast with Raspberry Syrup (page 51). In fact, Resistant Starch is in so many foods you crave that you'll have no trouble consuming the recommended amount.

Portion Control

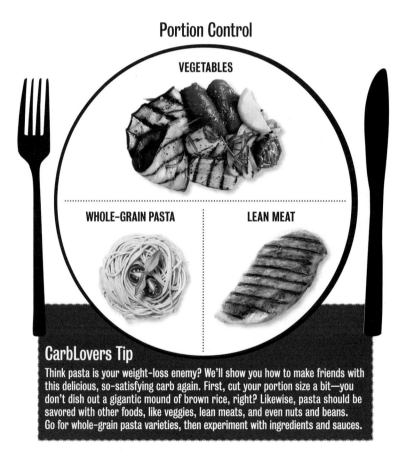

VEGETABLES

WHOLE-GRAIN PASTA

LEAN MEAT

CarbLovers Tip

Think pasta is your weight-loss enemy? We'll show you how to make friends with this delicious, so-satisfying carb again. First, cut your portion size a bit—you don't dish out a gigantic mound of brown rice, right? Likewise, pasta should be savored with other foods, like veggies, lean meats, and even nuts and beans. Go for whole-grain pasta varieties, then experiment with ingredients and sauces.

Top Resistant Starch Foods

FOOD	SERVING SIZE	GRAMS OF RESISTANT STARCH PER SERVING
Banana, slightly green	1 medium (7–8")	12.5
Banana, ripe	1 medium (7–8")	4.7
Oatmeal, raw/uncooked	½ cup	4.6
Beans, white, cooked/canned	½ cup	3.8
Lentils, cooked	½ cup	3.4
Potatoes, cooked and cooled	1 potato, 2.5" diameter	3.2
Plantain, cooked	½ cup, slices	2.7
Beans, garbanzo, cooked/canned	½ cup	2.1
Pasta, whole wheat, cooked	1 cup	2.0
Barley, pearled, cooked	½ cup	1.9
Pasta, white, cooked and cooled	1 cup	1.9
Beans, kidney, cooked/canned	½ cup	1.8
Potatoes, boiled (skin and flesh)	1 potato, 2.5" diameter	1.8
Rice, brown, cooked	½ cup	1.7
Beans, pinto, cooked/canned	½ cup	1.6
Peas, canned/frozen	½ cup	1.6
Pasta, white, cooked	1 cup	1.5
Beans, black, cooked/canned	½ cup	1.5

FOOD	SERVING SIZE	GRAMS OF RESISTANT STARCH PER SERVING
Millet, cooked	½ cup	1.5
Potatoes, baked (skin and flesh)	1 small	1.4
Bread, pumpernickel	1-oz slice	1.3
Corn polenta, cooked	½ cup	1.0
Yam, cooked	½ cup, cubes	1.0
Potato chips	1 oz	1.0
Cornflakes	1 cup	0.9
Bread, rye (whole)	1-oz slice	0.9
Puffed wheat	1¼ cups	0.9
Tortillas, corn	1 oz, 6" tortilla	0.8
English muffin	1 whole muffin	0.7
Bread, sourdough	1-oz slice	0.6
Crackers, rye crispbread	2 crispbreads	0.6
Oatmeal, cooked	1 cup	0.5
Bread, Italian	1-oz slice	0.3
Bread, whole grain	1-oz slice	0.3
Corn chips	1 oz	0.2
Crackers, crispbread (melba)	½ cup rounds	0.2

"I Lost Weight On CarbLovers"

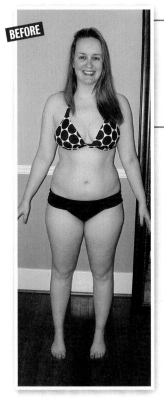

BEFORE

JEN WEST
Age: 31
Height: 5'10"
Weight before: 192
Weight after: 144
Pounds lost: 48

Biggest success moment: Slipping on size-8 jeans. The *Rachael Ray* show did a segment on *The CarbLovers Diet,* and I was one of the guests. So there I was in New York City about to be on national TV and fitting into these jeans, when I used to wear a size 16. I thought, "I can't believe this is my life."

Biggest challenge: Learning balance. I realized that a lot of my food issues had to do with control. If I'm not 100 percent in control, I tend to give up. I had to learn to lose my obsession with being perfect all of the time.

Favorite recipe: The Express Lunch Plate (page 70) was my go-to lunch for work. It was easy to throw together, and I could nibble on it when I was between tasks.

My job in a children's hospital is really stressful, and I relied on food to make me feel better. I never thought twice about hitting the drive-through or loading up on huge platefuls of pasta—then going back for seconds. When it came to food, I was a wild child. I had completely lost control. Being able to eat the things I love—like pasta and potatoes—is huge for me. *The CarbLovers Diet* keeps me feeling full. I'm not ravenous an hour or two after a meal, like I used to be. And I've learned to plan ahead for hunger emergencies. I keep Kashi TLC Oatmeal Raisin Flax cookies and pre-portioned bags of tortilla chips on hand if I'm on the go.

AFTER

I kept a daily blog (thejenwestquest.com) to track my weight-loss progress. My husband took weekly photos of me wearing a bikini to show how my body was changing. When I had a bad week, I definitely thought of photoshopping the image—but I chose honesty.

I told myself, "I will lose this weight, and I will learn to keep it off," and I set a goal for four months later. I was looking forward to wearing a black triangle-top bikini (and actually looking good in it), so we scheduled a cruise toward the end of the diet. It was such a victory to show off my new body!

I can't believe that I'm now the size I've wanted to be for such a long time. I was exercising before I started the diet—I even did a half-Ironman—so I was fit but fat. Now I'm training for a marathon, and my body is a lot lighter, so I've gotten so much faster. And I'm really confident that I can maintain this size and speed.

7-Day Kickstart Plan

THIS PLAN MAKES EATING THE *CARBLOVERS* WAY A TOTAL pleasure. In the first week, you'll lose up to six pounds while enjoying some of the most delicious meals and snacks you've ever tasted. And with every bite, you'll be learning a new way of eating that will get you to your weight-loss goal and keep you there—forever!

CarbLovers Tip

If you're the kind of eater who craves pasta in the morning and cereal at night, don't be afraid to substitute dinner for breakfast. Our daily plans will keep you on track, no matter how you choose your menu!

The *CarbLovers* Kickstart Plan is designed to keep you satisfied, so you won't be tempted to stray. We've provided simple recipes for when you feel like cooking and carefully selected prepared meals for when you just want something quick and easy. For the next week, you can follow our menus to the letter, or mix and match as your time and taste buds dictate. Either way, the 1,200 daily calories you'll be consuming will lead to only one outcome: rapid weight loss.

But before you begin, here are six simple rules to keep in mind.

1 Ditch the artificial sweeteners.

Studies suggest that the fake stuff, especially in diet sodas, doesn't promote weight loss and may even increase your craving for sugary foods (which make you pack on the pounds).

2 Prepare the same meals often.

The more you make something, the easier it is for you to re-create it. So get to know these recipes, which will be (we promise!) your best weight-loss buddies. Soon, you won't even need this book. You'll be able to shop for the right ingredients and create *CarbLovers* meals without our help, in your own kitchen, or wherever your travels take you.

③ Always eat your daily snack.

Snacks are important to this plan, because snacking prevents between-meal bingeing. Deciding when you eat your snack is up to you (most of our diet champs chose a few hours after lunch or an hour or two after dinner).

④ Don't skip meals.

The *CarbLovers* Kickstart Plan includes breakfast, lunch, dinner, and one snack a day. You must stick to this pattern to maintain your energy and keep hunger at bay.

⑤ Keep trigger foods out of your house.

By the end of the 21-Day *CarbLovers* Immersion Plan in Chapter 4, you'll be able to consume carbs with confidence. But you're not there yet. So rid your fridge and pantry of any food that makes you feel out of control. (For me, it's chocolate-chip-cookie dough!)

⑥ Don't drink liquid calories.

For the next seven days, you can drink water or coffee and tea—black, green, or herbal, without sweeteners, but with up to two teaspoons of low-fat milk—and my Secret Fat-Flushing Cocktail (below). Skip fruit juices, alcohol, and carbonated beverages (even diet sodas or sparkling water), which can make you look and feel bloated.

ELLEN'S SECRET FAT-FLUSHING COCKTAIL

This all-natural diet aid not only tastes great but may also help you burn off an extra 80 calories a day.

2 quarts (8 cups) brewed green tea
Juice from 1 orange
Juice from 1 lemon
Juice from 1 lime

Mix all ingredients together in a large pitcher.
Serve hot or iced; store it in the fridge for up to 3 days.

The Kickstart Shopping List

This grocery list will take you through the whole first week of recipes, and since it doesn't include a lot of pricey meats, it's economical, too! But on *CarbLovers*, you always have the option of choosing a grab-and-go meal instead of a homemade one, so you may need to modify this list to reflect your daily meal-plan choices.

PRODUCE

- Bananas, slightly green, 5 medium
- Tomatoes, 3 beefsteak, 3 cocktail (small oval)
- Onions, 2 medium
- Scallions, 1 bunch
- Zucchini, 2 large
- Baby spinach, 1 bag
- Kale, 1 bunch (will use 1 cup shredded)
- Baby carrots, 1 bag
- Large carrots, 1 bag
- Red grapes, 1 bunch (will use 2 cups)
- Red pepper
- Apples, 3 medium
- Garlic, 1 large head
- Fresh ginger, 1 small piece
- Basil, small bunch
- Strawberries, fresh (1 pint) or frozen (10-oz bag)
- Dried cranberries, 1 bag
- Red cabbage, 1 small head
- Ready-to-eat salad greens, 5 cups
- Romaine lettuce, 4 cups
- Avocado, 1
- Apple juice, 6.75-oz bottle
- Dried mango, 1/8 cup chopped

DAIRY/REFRIGERATED

- 1/2 gallon 1% milk
- Eggs, 1 dozen
- Sharp Cheddar cheese, 2 oz
- Cheddar cheese block, 16 oz
- Shredded part-skim mozzarella cheese (will use 1/2 cup)
- Grated fresh Parmesan cheese, about 2 cups
- Non-fat plain Greek yogurt, 32-oz container

- Yogurt, fat-free, 6-oz cup
- Light sour cream, 8-oz container
- Pepper jack cheese, 8-oz block
- Cheese sticks, 1 package

BREAD/GRAIN/CEREAL

- Rye bread, 1 loaf
- Pre-baked whole-wheat pizza crust, 1
- Wasa light rye crispbread crackers, 1 9.7-oz package
- Old-fashioned rolled oats, 42-oz canister
- Whole-wheat pita-bread rounds, 1 package
- Whole-wheat wraps/tortillas, 1 package of 8
- Cornflakes, 1 box
- Pumpernickel rolls, 1 bag (using 1)
- Whole-grain rotini, 1 box
- Corn tortillas, 12 (6" diameter)
- Puffed millet cereal, 1 box (using 3 cups)
- Wheat germ, small jar
- Brown rice, small box (using 1 1/2 cups cooked)
- Bow-tie or orecchiette pasta, 1 box
- Nature Valley Oats 'n Honey Crunchy Granola Bars, 1 box

MEAT/SEAFOOD

- Skinless, boneless chicken breast, 8 oz
- Canadian bacon, 8-oz package (using 2 slices)
- Lean, boneless ham, 4 oz
- Prosciutto, 2 thin slices
- Hummus, 10-oz container
- Natural chunky-style peanut butter, 12-oz jar

- Almond butter, 12-oz jar
- Applesauce, 8 oz
- Garbanzo beans, no added salt, 15½-oz can
- Black beans, no added salt, 2 15½-oz cans
- Chicken stock, low sodium, 1 32-oz container
- Kidney beans, 15½-oz can
- Cannellini beans, 15½-oz can
- Sliced almonds, ½ cup
- Chopped walnuts, ½ cup
- Chopped pecans, ½ cup
- Pumpkinseeds, ¼ cup

- Honey
- Whole-grain mustard
- Extra-virgin olive oil
- Canola oil
- Low-fat vinaigrette
- Cooking spray
- Sugar
- Salt
- All-purpose flour
- Whole-wheat pastry flour
- Baking powder
- Cinnamon
- Nutmeg
- Dried oregano
- Black pepper
- Salsa
- Maple syrup
- Dark sesame oil
- Soy sauce, low sodium
- Hot sauce
- Marinara sauce
- Dried mango, small package (will use ⅛ cup)

- Frozen peas, 10-oz box
- Frozen stir-fry vegetables, 1-lb bag (will use 4 cups)
- Medium shrimp, frozen or fresh, 3 oz (or 14)
- Raspberries, frozen or fresh, 1 cup

	MONDAY (DAY 1)
BREAKFAST	Banana Shake (page 57) OR 1 packet instant oatmeal + 1 TBSP chopped walnuts + 1 TBSP honey (optional)
LUNCH	Grilled Cheese & Tomato on Rye (page 73) + apple or pear OR EVOL Veggie Fajita Burrito
DINNER	Chicken Pasta Primavera (page 93) OR Kashi Mayan Harvest Bake + 2 cups salad greens with 2 TSP low-fat vinaigrette
SNACK	6 oz fat-free Greek yogurt + 2 TSP honey + 2 TBSP uncooked oats

	TUESDAY (DAY 2)	**WEDNESDAY (DAY 3)**
BREAKFAST	2 cups cornflakes + 1 cup 1% milk + 1 cup fresh or frozen strawberries OR Kashi TLC Chewy Granola Bar + fresh fruit (1 cup berries or 1 medium-size fruit)	Oatmeal-Cranberry Muffin* (page 52) + 1 TSP almond butter *(Banana-Nut Oatmeal, page 61, if you don't have time to bake muffins) OR Starbucks Apple Bran Muffin + hot green tea
LUNCH	Chicken Pita Sandwich (page 69) OR 1 Lean Pockets Whole Grain Turkey, Broccoli & Cheese (1 pocket) + 2 cups salad greens with 2 TBSP low-fat vinaigrette	Express Lunch Plate (page 70; may substitute 2-oz deli-sliced lean meat for egg) OR Subway 6" Turkey Breast Sandwich + Baked Lay's potato chips (1⅛-oz bag)
DINNER	Pizza with Prosciutto, Tomatoes & Parmesan Cheese (page 92) + 2 cups salad greens + 2 TSP low-fat vinaigrette OR Lean Cuisine Sun-Dried Tomato Pesto Chicken + 1 whole-wheat roll	Black Bean Tacos (page 95) OR Amy's Kitchen Light & Lean Spinach Lasagna
SNACK	10 baby carrots + 2 TBSP store-bought hummus	Trail mix: ½ cup cornflakes or multi-grain Cheerios + 2 TBSP dried cherries + 2 TBSP sliced almonds

	THURSDAY (DAY 4)	FRIDAY (DAY 5)
BREAKFAST	Banana & Almond Butter Toast (page 56; can substitute natural peanut butter) OR 2 whole-wheat frozen waffles + 2 TBSP almond or peanut butter	½ cup Granola with Pecans, Pumpkinseeds & Dried Mango* (page 48) + 6 oz fat-free Greek yogurt *(May substitute high-fiber breakfast cereal in place of granola) OR Kashi TLC Crunchy Granola Bars (2 bars per package) + 6 oz fat-free yogurt
LUNCH	Big Chopped Salad (page 79) OR Wendy's Apple Pecan Chicken Salad (half-size; other Wendy's salads allowed in half-servings: BLT Cobb and Baja)	Banana-Nut Elvis Wrap (page 72) + 10 baby carrots OR Bumble Bee tuna kit* + 1 pear *(Kit contains crackers and condiment, which are allowed)
DINNER	Three-Bean Soup with Canadian Bacon (page 67) + 1 whole-wheat or pumpernickel roll OR 2 cups Progresso High Fiber Homestyle Minestrone + 3 rye crispbread crackers	Pasta with Peas, Ham & Parmesan Cheese (page 94) OR Healthy Choice Café Steamers Chicken Pesto Classico
SNACK	½ cup red grapes + 1 (1-oz) cheese stick	Nature Valley Oats 'n Honey Crunchy Granola Bar (package contains 2 bars; both allowed)

	SATURDAY (DAY 6)	SUNDAY (DAY 7)
BREAKFAST	Spinach & Egg Breakfast Wrap with Avocado & Pepper Jack Cheese (page 53) **OR** Instant oatmeal (1 package) + 1 cup fresh berries or 1 medium fruit (mix instant oatmeal with 4 oz 1% milk, if desired)	2 cups cornflakes + 1 cup 1% milk + ½ sliced banana **OR** 2 frozen whole-wheat waffles + 1 TBSP almond or peanut butter
LUNCH	Lunch Shake (page 75) + 1 toasted whole-grain English muffin + 1 TBSP hummus **OR** Subway 6" Veggie Delight sandwich + Baked Lay's (1⅛-ounce bag)	Express Lunch Plate (page 70) **OR** Amy's Kitchen Southwestern Burrito + ¼ cup salsa
DINNER	Shrimp Stir-Fry with Ginger (page 88) **OR** Lean Cuisine Ginger Garlic Stir Fry with Chicken	Black Bean Tacos (page 95) **OR** Boca Burger on 1 toasted whole-grain bun + lettuce and mustard + 1 medium apple
SNACK	6 oz fat-free yogurt	10 baby carrots + 2 TBSP store-bought hummus

The 21-Day Immersion Plan

ONE WEEK INTO THE *CARBLOVERS* DIET, YOU CAN ALREADY see and feel the difference: Your clothes are a little looser, your skin is glowing, and you almost never feel hungry! Get ready to keep that slimmer you—and lose even more weight, if you want to—with The *CarbLovers* Immersion Plan, which takes our favorite quick-and-easy meals and adds even more delicious carbs.

For a full list of CarbLovers grab-and-go meals, see page 116!

We've increased the calories to about 1,600 a day by offering side dishes, an extra snack (some are even desserts!), and entrées with slightly bigger portions. As always, feel free to mix and match main dishes as you like, and choose as many grab-and-go options as you want. But for those who want to enjoy our recipes, we've included shopping lists for each week, on pages 26, 32, and 38.

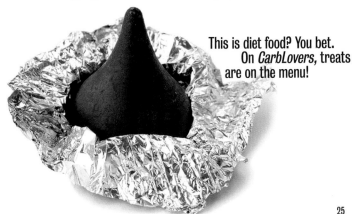

This is diet food? You bet. On *CarbLovers,* treats are on the menu!

Shopping List: Week 1

The following grocery list is for the *CarbLovers* recipes suggested in
Immersion Week 1. If you plan to include some or all ready-made options, you will
need to alter the list to fit your meal choices.

PRODUCE

- ❏ Fresh berries, 1 cup
- ❏ Strawberries, fresh (2 pt) or frozen (10-oz bag, using 3 cups)
- ❏ Bananas, slightly green, 2
- ❏ Large carrots, 1 bag
- ❏ Fresh spinach, 5-oz container
- ❏ Fresh chives, 1 bunch
- ❏ Arugula, 2 5-oz containers (using 6 cups)
- ❏ Red cabbage, 1 small head
- ❏ Mixed salad greens, 5 cups
- ❏ Red grapes, 1 bunch (using ½ cup)
- ❏ Yellow onions, 3
- ❏ Red onion, 1
- ❏ Red bell pepper, 1
- ❏ Shallot, 1 large
- ❏ Garlic, 1 bulb (using 8 cloves)
- ❏ Fresh parsley, 1 bunch
- ❏ Fresh cilantro, 1 bunch
- ❏ Romaine lettuce, 1 head
- ❏ Broccoli, 1 bunch (using 1 cup)
- ❏ Cocktail tomatoes, 1 carton
- ❏ Tomatoes, 3 large
- ❏ Roma tomatoes, 2
- ❏ Pear, 2
- ❏ Zucchini, 2 large
- ❏ Yukon gold potatoes, 1½-lb bag
- ❏ Lemons, 2
- ❏ Limes, 1
- ❏ Apples, 2
- ❏ Avocado, 1 large
- ❏ Jalapeño pepper, 1
- ❏ Butter lettuce, 1 small head
- ❏ Fresh basil leaves, 8

DAIRY/REFRIGERATED

- ❏ ½ gallon 1 % milk
- ❏ Low-fat plain Greek yogurt, 12 oz
- ❏ Parmigiano-Reggiano, ¾ cup finely grated
- ❏ Parmesan cheese, 5 oz
- ❏ Goat cheese, 4-oz log
- ❏ String cheese, 1 package (using 1 stick)
- ❏ Low-sodium Swiss cheese, 1 oz
- ❏ Cheddar cheese, 16-oz block
- ❏ Part-skim shredded mozzarella, ½ cup
- ❏ Feta-cheese crumbles, 2 TBSP
- ❏ Reduced-fat sour cream, 8-oz container (using 1 TBSP)
- ❏ Unsalted butter, using ½ cup
- ❏ Low-fat buttermilk, 1 qt (using ½ cup)
- ❏ Whipped cream, 1 cup
- ❏ Eggs, 1 dozen large (using 8 eggs)

BREAD/GRAIN/CEREAL

- ❏ Cornflakes, 1 box
- ❏ Puffed millet cereal, 3 cups
- ❏ Whole-wheat pita bread, 1 package
- ❏ Pumpernickel bread, 1 loaf
- ❏ Rye bread, 1 loaf
- ❏ Whole-wheat or pumpernickel rolls, 2
- ❏ Whole-wheat slider buns, 1 package
- ❏ Pre-baked whole-wheat pizza crust (such as Fabulous Flats), 1
- ❏ Nature Valley Peanut Butter Granola Bars, 1 box
- ❏ Thomas' Light Multi-Grain English Muffin, 1 package
- ❏ Whole-wheat spaghetti, ½ lb
- ❏ Whole-wheat breadcrumbs, ¼ cup
- ❏ Corn tortillas, 1 package (using 7)
- ❏ Kashi TLC Fruit & Grain Bars, 1 box
- ❏ Whole-grain rotini, 1 box
- ❏ Old-fashioned rolled oats, 44-oz canister
- ❏ Wasa Light Rye Crispbread, 1 box

MEAT/SEAFOOD

- ❏ Boneless, skinless chicken breast, 28 oz

- ❏ Ground bison, 1 lb
- ❏ Ground lean turkey breast, 1 lb
- ❏ Thinly sliced lean roast beef, 12 oz
- ❏ Lean deli ham, 1 oz
- ❏ Canadian bacon, 2 oz
- ❏ Prosciutto, 1 oz (8 thin slices)

PANTRY STAPLES

Many of these items were purchased for the *CarbLovers* Kickstart Plan and can already be found in your pantry at this point. Check first, and buy only what you need.

- ❏ Walnuts, 7 TBSP chopped
- ❏ Grainy mustard
- ❏ Balsamic vinegar
- ❏ Salt
- ❏ Pepper
- ❏ Applesauce (using ½ cup)
- ❏ Apple juice, 3 TBSP
- ❏ Natural peanut butter, 12-oz jar
- ❏ Garbanzo beans, 15-oz can
- ❏ Pinto beans, 15-oz can
- ❏ No-sodium-added black beans, 2 15-oz cans
- ❏ Kidney beans, 15-oz can
- ❏ Cannellini/white beans, 15-oz can
- ❏ Pecans, ⅓ cup chopped
- ❏ Pumpkinseeds, 2 TBSP
- ❏ Roasted red peppers, 1 jar
- ❏ Dried cranberries, 1 cup
- ❏ Dried cherries, 1 cup
- ❏ Dried mango, 3 TBSP chopped
- ❏ Vanilla extract
- ❏ Ground cinnamon
- ❏ Dried oregano
- ❏ Dried tarragon
- ❏ Dried dill
- ❏ Nutmeg
- ❏ Baking powder
- ❏ Baking soda
- ❏ Sugar
- ❏ Brown sugar, ¼ cup
- ❏ All-purpose flour
- ❏ Whole-wheat pastry flour

- ❏ Extra-virgin olive oil
- ❏ Canola oil
- ❏ Cider vinegar
- ❏ Low-fat balsamic vinaigrette
- ❏ Dijon mustard
- ❏ Crystallized ginger, ½ cup
- ❏ Cooking spray
- ❏ Low-sodium chicken stock, 32-oz container
- ❏ Marinara sauce, 24-oz jar (using ¾ cup)
- ❏ Salsa, 1 jar
- ❏ Maple syrup
- ❏ Crushed tomatoes, 26-oz can
- ❏ Honey
- ❏ Merlot wine, 1 bottle
- ❏ Hershey's Kisses Special Dark Mildly Sweet Chocolates, 12-oz bag (using 5 kisses)
- ❏ Baked Lay's potato chips, 1⅛-oz bag

FROZEN

- ❏ Frozen green beans, 16-oz bag (using 1 cup)
- ❏ Fruit sorbet, 1 pt (using ¾ cup)
- ❏ Frozen gnocchi, 14-oz bag
- ❏ Frozen whole-grain waffles, 1 box (using 2)
- ❏ Skinny Cow Low Fat Ice Cream Sandwiches, 6-pack (using 1)

CarbLovers Tip

To avoid overeating sweets, store chocolate and other treats in the freezer, so they're out of sight and out of mind!

	MONDAY (DAY 1)	TUESDAY (DAY 2)
BREAKFAST	2 cups cornflakes + 8 oz 1% milk + 1 cup berries OR Jimmy Dean D-Lights Turkey Sausage Whole Grain Bagel	Banana Shake (page 57) OR 2 Banana Nut VitaTops + 12 oz skim latte
LUNCH	Chicken Pita Sandwich (page 69) OR Amy's Brown Rice Bowl + 1 pumpernickel roll	Big Chopped Salad (page 79) + 1 toasted Thomas' Light Multi-Grain English Muffin OR Bumble Bee Sensations Seasoned Tuna Medley kit* + 1 medium apple *(Kit includes crackers and condiments, which are allowed)
DINNER	Gnocchi with Walnut-Arugula Pesto (page 89) + 1 whole-wheat or pumpernickel roll OR 2 cups Progresso High Fiber Homestyle Minestrone or Progresso High Fiber Creamy Tomato Basil + 2 rye crispbread crackers + 2 Mini Babybel Light cheese wheels	Spaghetti & Turkey Meatballs in Tomato Sauce (page 90) OR Amy's Baked Ziti Bowl + 2 cups salad greens + 2 TBSP low-fat vinaigrette
SNACK 1	Nature Valley Peanut Butter Crunchy Granola Bars* *(Package contains 2 bars; both bars allowed)	½ cup red grapes + 1 string cheese
SNACK 2	Skinny Cow Low Fat Ice Cream Sandwich	1 glass red wine (5 oz)

	WEDNESDAY (DAY 3)	THURSDAY (DAY 4)
BREAKFAST	2 whole-grain frozen waffles with 1 TBSP peanut butter or 1 TBSP maple syrup + 8 oz 1% milk OR Amy's Breakfast Scramble Wrap	Broccoli & Feta Omelet with Toast (page 50) OR Kashi TLC Chewy Granola Bar + fresh fruit (1 cup berries or melon, or 1 medium piece of fruit)
LUNCH	Roast Beef Pumpernickel Sandwich with Roasted Red Pepper, Arugula & Goat Cheese (page 74) OR Wendy's Apple Pecan Chicken Salad (half-serving) + 2 rye crispbread crackers	Grilled Cheese & Tomato on Rye (page 73) + 1 pear OR Amy's Indian Spinach Tofu Wrap + 1 apple
DINNER	Black Bean Tacos (page 95) OR Kashi Frozen Entrees Black Bean Mango + 2 cups salad greens + 2 TBSP low-fat vinaigrette	Chicken Pasta Primavera (page 93) OR Subway 6" Oven Roasted Chicken sandwich + Baked Lay's potato chips (1⅛ oz)
SNACK 1	6 oz plain low-fat Greek yogurt + 2 TBSP walnuts	White Bean & Herb Hummus with Crudités (page 115). Use store-bought hummus or make your own.
SNACK 2	¾ cup fruit sorbet	5 Hershey's Kisses Special Dark Mildly Sweet Chocolates

	FRIDAY (DAY 5)	SATURDAY (DAY 6)
BREAKFAST	½ cup Granola with Pecans, Pumpkinseeds & Dried Mango (page 48) + 6 oz plain low-fat Greek yogurt OR Panera Granola Parfait	Oatmeal-Cranberry Muffin* (page 52) + 1 TBSP almond or peanut butter + 1 cup 1% milk *(May also substitute Banana-Nut Oatmeal, page 61) OR Starbucks Apple Bran Muffin + hot green tea
LUNCH	Ham, Pear & Swiss Cheese Sandwich (page 80) + Baked Lay's potato chips (1⅛ oz) OR 1 Lean Pocket Whole Grain Turkey, Broccoli & Cheese + 1 banana	Express Lunch Plate (page 70) OR Subway 6" Turkey Sandwich + Baked Lay's potato chips (1⅛ oz)
DINNER	Seared Chicken Breasts with French Potato Salad (page 104) OR 2 cups Progresso High Fiber Homestyle Minestrone soup + 2 rye crispbread crackers + 2 Mini Babybel Light cheese wheels	Bison Sliders with Guacamole (page 98) OR Boca Burger with sliced tomato, lettuce, onion, and mustard on a toasted whole-grain bun + 12 Alexia Sweet Potato Julienne Fries
SNACK 1	Kashi TLC Fruit & Grain Bar	Cheddar & Apple Melt (page 114)
SNACK 2	½ cup Banana Ice Cream (page 109)	1 glass red wine (5 oz)

	SUNDAY (DAY 7)
BREAKFAST	Cherry-Ginger Scone* (page 58) *(May substitute Coconut French Toast with Raspberry Syrup, page 51) OR Dunkin' Donuts Ham, Egg White & Cheese on Wheat English Muffin
LUNCH	Three-Bean Soup with Canadian Bacon (page 66) + 1 whole-wheat or pumpernickel roll OR Kashi Lemongrass Coconut Chicken + 1 whole-wheat or pumpernickel roll
DINNER	Pizza with Prosciutto, Tomatoes & Parmesan Cheese (page 92) + 2 cups salad greens + 2 TBSP low-fat vinaigrette OR Amy's Southwestern Burrito + ¼ cup salsa + 2 TBSP low-fat sour cream and 5 multi-grain tortilla chips (such as Food Should Taste Good)
SNACK 1	1 TBSP almond or peanut butter spread on 2 Wasa Light Rye Crispbread crackers
SNACK 2	Merlot Strawberries with Whipped Cream (page 106)

BANANA SHAKE:
RECIPE ON PAGE 57.

Shopping List: Week 2

The following grocery list is for the *CarbLovers* recipes suggested in Immersion Week 2. If you plan to include some or all ready-made options, you will need to alter the list to fit your meal choices.

PRODUCE

- ❏ Berries, 1½ cups
- ❏ Bananas, slightly green, 4
- ❏ Lemons, 2
- ❏ Arugula, 9 cups
- ❏ Grape tomatoes, ½ cup
- ❏ Lime, 1
- ❏ Fresh ginger, 1 small piece
- ❏ Mixed salad greens, 2 cups
- ❏ Coleslaw mix, 14-oz bag (using 3 cups)
- ❏ Fresh strawberries, 2 pt (using 3 cups)
- ❏ Baby carrots, 1-lb bag
- ❏ Onions, 3
- ❏ Scallions, 1 bunch
- ❏ Parsley, 1 bunch
- ❏ Pear, 1
- ❏ Garlic, 1 bulb (using 6 cloves)
- ❏ Fresh cilantro, 1 bunch
- ❏ Fresh mint, 1 bunch
- ❏ Red grapes, 1 bunch
- ❏ Blueberries, 1 cup
- ❏ Apple, 1
- ❏ Green leaf lettuce, 1 head
- ❏ Roma tomato, 1
- ❏ Carrots (whole), small bag
- ❏ Avocado, 1
- ❏ Raspberries, 1 pt
- ❏ Zucchini, 1 large
- ❏ Idaho potatoes, 4
- ❏ Broccoli florets, 2 cups fresh or 1 1-oz frozen package

DAIRY/REFRIGERATED

- ❏ Mini Babybel Light cheese wheels, 1 bag of 6 (using 2)
- ❏ Low-fat cottage cheese, ½ cup
- ❏ Eggs, 1 dozen large (using 4)
- ❏ ½ gallon 1% milk

- ❏ Parmesan cheese, 2 cups grated
- ❏ Plain low-fat Greek yogurt, 32-oz container (using 3¼ cups)
- ❏ Part-skim ricotta cheese, ¼ cup
- ❏ Sharp Cheddar cheese (using 1 slice)
- ❏ Goat cheese, 4-oz log
- ❏ Whipped cream, 1¼ cups
- ❏ Reduced-fat extra-sharp Cheddar, 4 oz shredded

BREAD/GRAIN/CEREAL

- ❏ Rye bread, 4 slices
- ❏ Corn tortillas, 12 (6")
- ❏ Nature Valley Crunchy Granola Bars, 1 box
- ❏ Cornflakes, 1 box
- ❏ Whole-wheat wraps, 4 10" wraps and 4 6" wraps
- ❏ Pearled barley, 3¾ cups uncooked
- ❏ Whole-grain pita, 1
- ❏ Wasa Light Rye Crispbread, 1 box (using 2 crackers)
- ❏ Multi-grain tortilla chips, 1 bag
- ❏ Old-fashioned rolled oats, 42-oz canister
- ❏ Kashi TLC bars, 1 box (using 1)
- ❏ Pumpernickel bread, 1 loaf
- ❏ Pumpernickel roll
- ❏ Quick-cooking brown rice, 1 cup uncooked
- ❏ Odwalla Banana Nut Bar, 1, or Odwalla Blueberry Swirl Bar, 1
- ❏ Puffed millet cereal, 3 cups
- ❏ Instant steel-cut oats, 42-oz canister (using 5¾ cups)
- ❏ Whole-wheat fusilli pasta, ½ pound dried
- ❏ Sourdough bread, 4 (½") slices

MEAT/SEAFOOD

- ❏ Skinless salmon fillets, 4 4-oz fillets
- ❏ Tilapia fillets, 1½ lb

- Pork tenderloin, 1 lb
- Grilled chicken breast, 8 oz
- Boneless, skinless chicken, 2 lb
- Thinly sliced lean roast beef, 12 oz
- Low-fat Italian sausage, 2 links (6 oz)
- Canadian bacon, 2 2-oz slices

PANTRY STAPLES

- Salt
- Pepper
- Toasted sesame seeds, 1 TBSP
- Toasted sesame oil
- Apricot jam, 2 TBSP
- Dried apricots, ½ cup
- Apple juice, 3 TBSP
- White beans, 15-oz can
- Low-sodium black beans, 2 15-oz cans
- Low-sodium cannellini beans, 2 15-oz cans
- Kidney beans, 15-oz can
- Chunky natural-style peanut butter 12-oz jar
- Chopped pecans, ¾ cup
- Pumpkinseeds, 2 TBSP
- Chopped walnuts, ¼ cup
- Honey
- Extra-virgin olive oil
- Dijon mustard, 1 jar
- Dark sesame oil, 1 jar
- Low-sodium soy sauce
- Cinnamon, ground
- Cumin
- Dried oregano
- Fire-roasted tomatoes, 15-oz can
- Hominy, 15-oz can
- Diced green chiles, 1 TBSP (small can)
- Slivered almonds, 3 TBSP
- Vanilla extract
- Maple syrup
- Merlot wine, 1 bottle
- Cooking spray
- Roasted red peppers, 1 jar
- Balsamic vinegar

- Semisweet chocolate chips, 12-oz bag (using 6 TBSP)
- Canola oil
- Chili flakes
- Hershey's Special Dark Miniatures, 11-oz bag (using 3)
- Light brown sugar
- Low-fat balsamic vinaigrette, 1 bottle
- Chili powder
- Diced tomatoes, 26-oz can
- Low-sodium chicken stock, 2 32-oz containers
- All-purpose flour
- Cayenne pepper
- Dried mango, 3 TBSP (chopped)
- Shredded coconut, 2 TBSP
- Marinated artichoke hearts, 12-oz jar
- Black olives, 12 olives
- Tuna in water, 3 oz

FROZEN

- Frozen stir-fry vegetables, 2 16-oz bags
- Large shrimp, frozen, cooked, 1 lb (using 3 oz)

	MONDAY (DAY 8)	**TUESDAY (DAY 9)**
BREAKFAST	Banana Shake (page 57) OR 1 packet instant oatmeal + 2 TBSP chopped walnuts + ½ TSP ground cinnamon	2 cups cornflakes + 8 oz 1% milk + 1 cup berries OR Kashi Chewy TLC bar and fresh fruit (1 cup berries or melon, or 1 medium piece of fruit)
LUNCH	Arugula Salad with Lemon-Dijon Dressing (page 68) OR Panera Grilled Chicken Caesar Salad* *(Order dressing on the side, and use sparingly)	Banana-Nut Elvis Wrap (page 72) + 10 baby carrots OR 2 cups Progresso High Fiber Homestyle Minestrone or Progresso High Fiber Creamy Tomato Basil Soup + 2 Wasa Light Rye Crispbread crackers
DINNER	Fish Tacos with Sesame-Ginger Slaw (page 103) OR Lean Cuisine Salmon with Basil + 1 cup Birds Eye Steamfresh Broccoli, Cauliflower & Carrots	Roasted Pork Tenderloin with Apricot-Barley Pilaf (page 96) OR Wendy's BLT Cobb Salad, half-size
SNACK 1	Nature Valley Peanut Butter Crunchy Granola Bar or Clif Crunch Granola Bar (Package contains 2 bars; both bars are allowed)	6 oz low-fat Greek yogurt with 2 TSP honey
SNACK 2	2 Dark Chocolate & Oat Clusters (page 111)	Warm Pear with Cinnamon Ricotta (page 110)

	WEDNESDAY (DAY 10)	**THURSDAY (DAY 11)**
BREAKFAST	Blueberry Oat Pancakes with Maple Yogurt (page 64) OR 1 Lean Pocket Applewood Bacon, Egg & Cheese	Sharp Cheddar & Egg on Rye (page 60) OR 2 frozen whole-grain waffles + 1 TBSP almond or peanut butter + 8 oz 1% milk
LUNCH	Red Grape & Tuna Salad Pita (page 76) OR Amy's Spinach Feta in a Pocket + ½ cup grapes	Roast Beef Pumpernickel Sandwich with Roasted Red Pepper, Arugula & Goat Cheese (page 74) OR Così Hummus & Fresh Veggies Sandwich + 1 apple
DINNER	Hearty Chicken Posole Stew (page 86) + 5 multi-grain tortilla chips OR Healthy Choice Oven Roasted Chicken	Shrimp Stir-Fry with Ginger (page 88) + 2 cups salad greens with 2 TBSP low-fat vinaigrette OR Lean Cuisine Ginger Garlic Stir Fry with Chicken + 2 cups salad greens with 2 TBSP low-fat vinaigrette
SNACK 1	2 Mini Babybel Light cheese wheels + 2 Wasa Light Rye crispbread crackers	Odwalla Blueberry Swirl Bar or Odwalla Banana Nut Bar
SNACK 2	1 glass red wine (5 oz)	Chocolate-Dipped Banana Bites* (page 113) *(May substitute 1 cup fresh strawberries or ¼ cup dried apricots in place of banana)

	FRIDAY (DAY 12)	SATURDAY (DAY 13)
BREAKFAST	½ cup Granola with Pecans, Pumpkinseeds & Dried Mango (page 48) + 6 oz plain low-fat Greek yogurt OR 1 cup Fiber One Original cereal + 8 oz 1% milk + 1 cup berries	Steel-Cut Oatmeal with Salted Caramel Topping* (page 62) *(May substitute Banana-Nut Oatmeal, page 61) OR Subway Egg (White) & Cheese Muffin Melt
LUNCH	Gnocchi with Walnut-Arugula Pesto (page 89) OR Wendy's Apple Pecan Chicken Salad, half-size	Black Bean, Avocado, Brown Rice & Chicken Wrap* (page 81) *(Make it faster! Use instant or quick-cooking brown rice) OR Amy's Brown Rice Bowl + 10 baby carrots + 1 pumpernickel roll
DINNER	Honey & Sesame-Glazed Salmon with Confetti Barley Salad (page 84) OR Healthy Choice Café Steamers Chicken Margherita	Sausage, Tomato, White Bean & Corkscrew Pasta Toss (page 100) OR P.F. Chang's Buddha's Feast, steamed, with brown rice
SNACK 1	Antipasto platter: 12 black olives, ½ cup marinated artichoke hearts, and ½ bottle roasted red peppers (sliced)	6 oz low-fat yogurt + 2 TBSP Granola with Pecans, Pumpkinseeds & Dried Mango (page 48) or other low-fat granola
SNACK 2	3 Hershey's Special Dark Miniatures	1 glass red wine (5 oz)

	SUNDAY (DAY 14)
BREAKFAST	Coconut French Toast with Raspberry Syrup (page 51) OR Panera Granola Parfait
LUNCH	Three-Bean Soup with Canadian Bacon (page 66) + pumpernickel roll OR Subway 6" Veggie Delight Sandwich + Baked Lay's potato chips (1⅛ oz)
DINNER	Broccoli & Cheese-Stuffed Baked Potato (page 101) OR 2 cups Progresso High Fiber Creamy Tomato Basil soup + 1 toasted Thomas' Light Multi-Grain English Muffin
SNACK 1	Kashi TLC bar + ½ cup red grapes
SNACK 2	Merlot Strawberries with Whipped Cream (page 106)

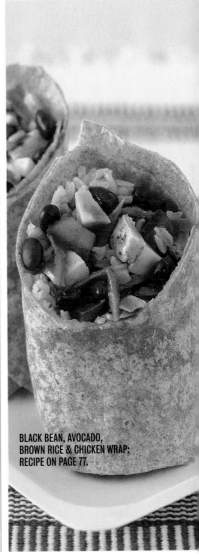

BLACK BEAN, AVOCADO, BROWN RICE & CHICKEN WRAP; RECIPE ON PAGE 77.

Shopping List: Week 3

The following grocery list is for the *CarbLovers* recipes suggested in Immersion Week 3. If you plan to include some or all ready-made options, you will need to alter the list to fit your meal choices.

PRODUCE

- ❑ Berries, 1 cup
- ❑ Bananas, slightly green, 5
- ❑ Scallions, 2 bunches
- ❑ Tomatoes, beefsteak, 2
- ❑ Mixed salad greens, 1 bag
- ❑ Red cabbage, ½ cup shredded
- ❑ Baby spinach, 1 lb
- ❑ Green leaf lettuce, 4 leaves
- ❑ Avocados, 3
- ❑ Red onion, 1
- ❑ Roma tomatoes, 3
- ❑ Butter lettuce, 1 head
- ❑ Cilantro, 1 bunch
- ❑ Jalapeño pepper, 1
- ❑ Oranges, 2
- ❑ Red pepper, 1
- ❑ Limes, 2
- ❑ Grape tomatoes, 1 pt
- ❑ Apples, 2
- ❑ Zucchini, 1 large
- ❑ Baby carrots, 1 small bag
- ❑ Green beans, 1½ cups
- ❑ Green bell pepper, 1
- ❑ Romaine lettuce, 1 head
- ❑ Carrots, 1 bag
- ❑ Cucumber, 1
- ❑ Blueberries, 1 cup
- ❑ Yukon gold potatoes, 1½ pounds
- ❑ Fresh parsley, 1 bunch
- ❑ Shallot, 1 large
- ❑ Fresh tarragon, 1 small bunch
- ❑ Lemons, 3
- ❑ Red grapes, 1 small bunch
- ❑ Fresh mint, 1 TBSP chopped
- ❑ Onion, 1
- ❑ Garlic, 1 bulb (using 1 clove)

DAIRY/REFRIGERATED

- ❑ ½ gallon 1% milk
- ❑ Hummus, 4 TBSP
- ❑ Mini Babybel Light cheese wheels, 1 bag
- ❑ Reduced-fat Cheddar-cheese slices, 8 oz
- ❑ Grated Parmesan cheese, 1 cup + 1 TBSP
- ❑ Pepper jack cheese, 4 oz shredded
- ❑ Reduced-fat sour cream, 8 oz container (using 5 oz)
- ❑ Low-fat plain Greek yogurt, 7-oz container
- ❑ Brie cheese, 1 oz
- ❑ Cheddar cheese, ¼ cup shredded
- ❑ Feta cheese, 2 oz crumbled (using 1 TBSP)
- ❑ Low-fat cottage cheese, 4 oz
- ❑ Goat cheese, 4-oz log
- ❑ Unsalted butter, 1 stick
- ❑ Part-skim ricotta cheese, ¼ cup
- ❑ String cheese, 1 package
- ❑ Swiss cheese, 2 oz
- ❑ Shredded potatoes, 1 package refrigerated (such as Simply Potatoes)
- ❑ Eggs, 2 dozen large

BREAD/GRAIN/CEREAL

- ❑ Rye bread, 1 loaf
- ❑ Pearled barley, ¾ cup uncooked
- ❑ Old-fashioned rolled oats, 14-oz canister
- ❑ Whole-wheat tortillas, 4
- ❑ Whole-wheat slider buns, 8
- ❑ Whole-wheat wraps, 4 8" wraps and 4 10" wraps
- ❑ Kashi TLC Original 7 Grain Snack Crackers, 1 box
- ❑ Brown rice, 1½ cups uncooked
- ❑ Corn tortillas, 4 (6")

- Cornflakes, 1 box
- Puffed-wheat cereal, 1 box
- Whole-wheat orecchiette pasta, 8 oz dried
- Whole-grain hamburger buns, 2
- Pumpernickel bread, 1 loaf
- Whole-grain pita, 1

MEAT/SEAFOOD

- Grilled chicken breast, 8 oz
- Salmon, 4 4-oz fillets
- Ground bison, 1 lb
- Lean boneless ham, 4 oz
- Boneless, skinless chicken breast (4 5-oz breasts)
- Thinly sliced lean roast beef, 12 oz
- Canadian bacon, 1 package (using 1 oz)
- Scallops, fresh or frozen, 1 lb (about 16)
- Lean ground sirloin, 6 oz

PANTRY STAPLES

- Tarragon
- Flour
- Salt
- Pepper
- Grainy mustard, 4 TBSP
- Balsamic vinegar
- Black beans, 2 15-oz cans
- White beans, 15-oz can
- Kidney beans, 15-oz can
- Dried cranberries, small package (using 1 TBSP)
- Cumin
- Dried oregano
- Extra-virgin olive oil
- Vanilla extract
- Maple syrup
- Dijon mustard, 1 small jar
- Cider vinegar, 1 TBSP
- Roasted red peppers, 1 jar
- Black olives, 1 small can or 1 small container from salad bar
- Dried dates, 8
- Marinated artichoke hearts, 1 can
- Sugar
- Fine corn meal
- Chili powder
- Curry powder
- Semisweet chocolate chips, ¼ cup
- Yellow corn, 11-oz can
- Hershey's Kisses Special Dark Mildly Sweet Chocolates, 1 small bag
- Salsa, 1 small jar
- Dried dill
- Red wine, 1 bottle
- 70% dark chocolate, 3 oz
- Sesame seeds, 1 TBSP toasted
- Honey
- Low-sodium soy sauce
- Chili flakes
- Cooking spray
- Low-fat balsamic vinaigrette, 1 bottle
- Hot sauce, 1 bottle
- Natural-style peanut butter, 12-oz jar
- Luna Bar, 1
- Slivered almonds, 3 TBSP
- Dried cherries, 2 TBSP
- Shredded coconut, 2 TBSP
- Almond butter, 12-oz jar
- Tuna in water, 1 can

FROZEN

- Frozen peas, 10-oz package
- Skinny Cow Low Fat Ice Cream Sandwiches, 6-pack (using 2)

CarbLovers Tip

Have extra time this weekend? Whip up a batch of our amazing Cherry–Ginger Scones and freeze them to enjoy all week!

	MONDAY (DAY 15)	**TUESDAY (DAY 16)**
BREAKFAST	Banana Shake (page 57) OR Amy's Breakfast Scramble Wrap	Spinach & Egg Breakfast Wrap with Avocado & Pepper Jack Cheese (page 53) OR 1 CranBran VitaTop Muffin Top + 1 TSP almond or peanut butter + 8 oz 1% milk
LUNCH	Grilled Cheese & Tomato on Rye (page 73) + 1 apple OR Bumble Bee Sensations Seasoned Tuna Medley kit* + 1 apple *(Kit includes crackers and condiments, which are allowed)	Big Chopped Salad (page 79) OR Amy's Black Bean Enchilada Whole Meal with Spanish Rice & Beans
DINNER	Honey & Sesame-Glazed Salmon with Confetti Barley Salad (page 84) OR Healthy Choice Café Steamers Grilled Basil Chicken	Bison Sliders with Guacamole (page 98) OR Kashi Chicken Florentine + 2 cups mixed greens + 2 TBSP low-fat vinaigrette
SNACK 1	2 Mini Babybel Light cheese wheels + 7 Kashi TLC Crackers Original 7 Grain * *(May substitute 4 Wheat Thins or Triscuits)	Luna Bar
SNACK 2	Skinny Cow Low Fat Ice Cream Sandwich	2 Dark Chocolate & Oat Clusters (page 111)

	WEDNESDAY (DAY 17)	THURSDAY (DAY 18)
BREAKFAST	Banana & Almond Butter Toast (page 56; can substitute natural peanut butter) OR 2 frozen whole-grain waffles + 1 TBSP almond or peanut butter	Banana Shake (page 57) OR Kashi TLC bar + 12-oz skim latte
LUNCH	Black Bean & Zucchini Quesadillas (page 77) OR Healthy Choice Honey Balsamic Chicken + 2 cups salad greens with 2 TBSP low-fat vinaigrette	Curried Egg Salad Sandwich (page 78) OR Kashi Frozen Entrees Lemongrass Coconut Chicken + Wasa Light Rye Crispbread crackers
DINNER	Pasta with Peas, Ham & Parmesan Cheese (page 94) OR Kashi Frozen Entrees Veggie Chana Masala + ½ cup baby carrots	Pan-Seared Scallops with Southwestern Rice Salad (page 102) OR Healthy Choice Café Steamers Lemon Garlic Chicken and Shrimp + 1 whole-wheat or pumpernickel roll
SNACK 1	Trail mix: ½ cup cornflakes, 2 TBSP sliced almonds, and 2 TBSP dried cherries	1 small sliced apple with 1 oz Brie cheese
SNACK 2	2 Coconut-Date Truffles (page 108)	5 Hershey's Kisses Special Dark Mildly Sweet Chocolates

	FRIDAY (DAY 19)	SATURDAY (DAY 20)
BREAKFAST	2 cups cornflakes + 1 cup 1% milk + 1 cup berries OR 1 packet instant oatmeal + 2 TSP chopped walnuts	Blueberry Oat Pancakes with Maple Yogurt (page 64) OR Amy's Breakfast Burrito + 1 navel orange
LUNCH	Banana-Nut Elvis Wrap (page 72) + 10 baby carrots OR Lean Cuisine Sun Dried Tomato Pesto Chicken + 1 whole-wheat or pumpernickel roll	Roast Beef Pumpernickel Sandwich with Roasted Red Pepper, Arugula & Goat Cheese (page 74) OR 1 Amy's Black Bean Vegetable Enchilada + ¼ cup salsa + 5 multi-grain tortilla chips + 1 apple
DINNER	Grilled Burger & Three-Bean Salad (page 87) OR Amy's Chili & Cornbread Whole Meal	Seared Chicken Breasts with French Potato Salad (page 104) OR Healthy Choice Café Steamers Grilled Vegetables Mediterranean + 1 whole-wheat or pumpernickel roll
SNACK 1	Hummus with feta and dill: Top 4 TBSP store-bought hummus with 1 TBSP feta cheese and ⅛ TSP dried dill; serve with 1 cup sliced cucumbers	Antipasto platter: 12 black olives, ½ cup marinated artichoke hearts, and ½ bottle roasted red peppers (sliced)
SNACK 2	1 glass red wine (5 oz)	Chocolate-Orange Spoonbread (page 112)

	SUNDAY (DAY 21)
BREAKFAST	Potato-Crusted Spinach Quiche (page 54) **OR** Aunt Jemima Scrambled Eggs and Bacon with Hash Brown Potatoes
LUNCH	Black Bean, Avocado, Brown Rice & Chicken Wrap* (page 81) *(Make it faster! Use instant or quick-cooking brown rice) **OR** Subway 6" Oven Roasted Chicken Sandwich + Baked Lay's potato chips (1⅛ oz)
DINNER	Red Grape & Tuna Salad Pita (page 76) **OR** Boca Burger on toasted bun with lettuce, tomato, and mustard + 12 Alexia Sweet Potato Julienne Fries
SNACK 1	String cheese + apple
SNACK 2	Skinny Cow Low Fat Ice Cream Sandwich

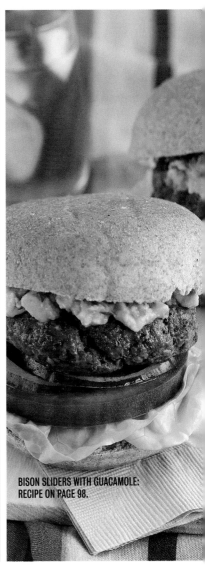

BISON SLIDERS WITH GUACAMOLE: RECIPE ON PAGE 98.

"I Lost Weight On CarbLovers"

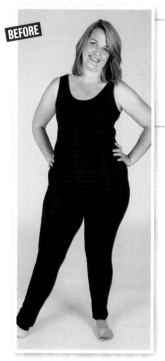

BEFORE

STARLA WILKINS
Age: 35
Height: 5'5"
Weight before: 176
Weight after: 146
Pounds lost: 30

Biggest success moment: As I was dropping my son Greyson off at a birthday party, he looked at me and said, "Oh, Mommy, you look really skinny in that sweater." The fact that a 9-year-old boy would notice just felt incredible.

Biggest challenge: Giving up soda and mindless snacking. Every afternoon I would reach for a soda. Then I would binge-snack as I was cooking dinner. I'd wander over to my pantry and eat cookies, chips, chocolaty granola bars—you name it, I ate it. But I've come this far—I can't go back now.

Favorite recipe: All the recipes are fantastic, because the whole family loves them. My kids ask for the Banana Shake (page 57) for breakfast.

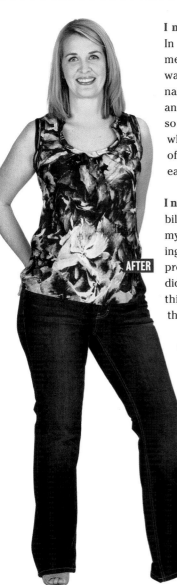

AFTER

I never had weight issues growing up. In high school, my classmates teased me about being so skinny. That's why it was so hard for me to get all the pregnancy weight off—I didn't know how. I'm an on-the-go mom of three young boys, so my eating strategy was "Eat whatever— whenever you can!" I never planned any of my meals. So when I had a chance to eat, I'd snack like crazy.

I never feel like I'm on a diet. My grocery bill hasn't gone up. I still cook dinner for my family every night, only now we're eating brown rice instead of white, and lean protein instead of fried chicken. My kids didn't have a clue about the switch. Everything tastes great, so they didn't notice that we were eating differently.

CarbLovers **taught me to sit down every Sunday night and plan out my menus for the week.** Since I always know what I'm going to prepare, I never have to think about what to make when I'm hungry. I never stand in front of my refrigerator feeling tempted by the bad stuff. My whole family is healthier because we all eat the *CarbLovers* recipes together, and I've switched to healthier snacks. There isn't any guesswork, and everything tastes so good that I never have a chance to slip up.

The CarbLovers Recipe Collection

DINNER

- Bison Sliders with Guacamole, page 98
- Black Bean Tacos, page 95
- Broccoli & Cheese-Stuffed Baked Potato, page 101
- Chicken Pasta Primavera, page 93
- Fish Tacos with Sesame-Ginger Slaw, page 103
- Gnocchi with Walnut-Arugula Pesto, page 89
- Grilled Burger & Three-Bean Salad, page 87
- Hearty Chicken Posole Stew, page 86
- Honey & Sesame-Glazed Salmon with Confetti Barley Salad, page 84
- Orecchiette with White Beans & Pesto, page 97
- Pan-Seared Scallops with Southwestern Rice Salad, page 102
- Pasta with Peas, Ham & Parmesan Cheese, page 94
- Pizza with Prosciutto, Tomatoes & Parmesan Cheese, page 92
- Roasted Pork Tenderloin with Apricot-Barley Pilaf, page 96
- Sausage, Tomato, White Bean & Corkscrew Pasta Toss, page 100
- Seared Chicken Breasts with French Potato Salad, page 104
- Shrimp Stir-Fry with Ginger, page 88
- Spaghetti & Turkey Meatballs in Tomato Sauce, page 90

DESSERTS

- Banana Ice Cream, page 109
- Chocolate-Dipped Banana Bites, page 113
- Chocolate-Orange Spoonbread, page 112
- Coconut-Date Truffles, page 108
- Dark Chocolate & Oat Clusters, page 111
- Merlot Strawberries with Whipped Cream, page 106
- Warm Pear with Cinnamon Ricotta, page 110

SNACKS

- Antipasto Platter, page 114
- Brie & Apple Slices, page 114
- Cheddar & Apple Melt, page 114
- Greek Yogurt with Orange Marmalade & Walnuts, page 114
- Honey-Curried Yogurt Dip with Carrots & Broccoli, page 114
- Hummus with Feta & Dill, page 114
- Pistachio & Dried Cherry Crostini, page 114
- Salmon & Cream Cheese Bites, page 114
- Trail Mix, page 114
- White Bean & Herb Hummus with Crudités, page 115

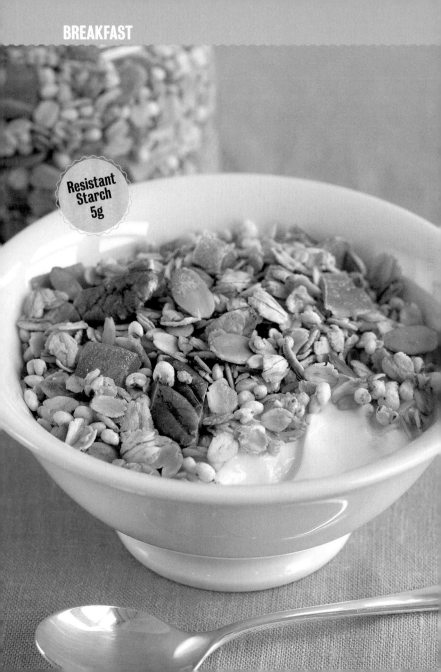

Resistant
Starch
5g

Granola with Pecans, Pumpkinseeds & Dried Mango

PREP: 5 MINUTES
COOK: 25 MINUTES
TOTAL TIME: 30 MINUTES
MAKES: 6 SERVINGS (3 CUPS TOTAL)

- 3 cups old-fashioned rolled oats
- 3 cups puffed millet cereal
- ⅓ cup lightly toasted chopped pecans
- 2 tablespoons pumpkinseeds
- 1 tablespoon canola oil
- 5 tablespoons maple syrup
- 3 tablespoons apple juice or apple cider
- 1 teaspoon vanilla extract
- ¼ teaspoon salt
- 3 tablespoons chopped dried mango

1. Preheat oven to 350°.
2. Line a large rimmed baking sheet with parchment paper and reserve.
3. Combine oats, puffed millet, pecans, and pumpkinseeds in a large bowl.
4. Whisk together canola oil, maple syrup, apple juice, vanilla, and salt in a small bowl and toss with dry ingredients.
5. Spread on a large parchment-lined baking sheet, and bake until golden brown, stirring occasionally, 20–25 minutes.
6. Remove from oven, let cool completely, and toss with dried mango.

Serving size: ½ cup granola | Calories 331; Fat 11g (sat 1g, mono 5g, poly 4g); Cholesterol 0mg; Protein 8g; Carbohydrate 52g; Sugars 14g; Fiber 5g; RS 5g; Sodium 54mg

Crunchy nuts and chewy mango give a flavor-packed start to your day.

Broccoli & Feta Omelet with Toast

PREP: 5 MINUTES
COOK: 10 MINUTES
TOTAL TIME: 15 MINUTES
MAKES: 1 SERVING

Cooking spray
1 cup chopped broccoli
2 large eggs, whisked
2 tablespoons feta cheese, crumbled
¼ teaspoon dried dill
2 slices rye bread, toasted

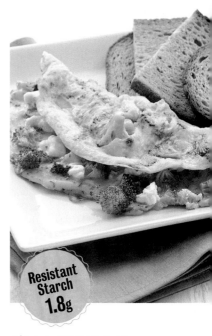

1. Heat a nonstick skillet over medium heat. Coat pan with cooking spray. Add broccoli, and cook 3 minutes.

2. Combine eggs, feta, and dill in a small bowl. Add egg mixture to pan. Cook 3–4 minutes; fold in half with a spatula, and cook 2 more minutes or until cooked through. Serve with toast.

Resistant Starch
1.8g

Serving size: 1 omelet and 2 pieces toast | Calories 390; Fat 19g (sat 6g, mono 5g, poly 2g); Cholesterol 440mg; Protein 23g; Carbohydrate 35g; Sugars 5g; Fiber 6g; RS 1.8g; Sodium 550mg

Coconut French Toast with Raspberry Syrup

PREP: 5 MINUTES
COOK: 10 MINUTES
TOTAL TIME: 15 MINUTES
MAKES: 2 SERVINGS

- 2 large eggs
- ½ cup 1% low-fat milk
- 1 teaspoon vanilla extract
- 4 (½-inch-thick) slices sourdough bread
- 2 tablespoons shredded coconut
  Cooking spray
- 1 cup raspberries
- 2 tablespoons pure maple syrup

1. In a large bowl, whisk together eggs, milk, and vanilla.
2. Lightly dip bread slices in egg mixture; pat shredded coconut onto both sides of bread.
3. Heat a large nonstick skillet over medium heat. Coat pan with cooking spray. Add bread slices; cook 4 minutes on each side or until golden.
4. Combine raspberries and maple syrup in a small microwave-safe bowl. Microwave at HIGH 30 seconds. Serve over French toast.

Serving size: 2 pieces French toast and 4 tablespoons syrup | Calories 410; Fat 12g (sat 5g, mono 2.5g, poly 1.5g); Cholesterol 215mg; Protein 16g; Carbohydrate 58g; Sugars 20g; Fiber 6g; RS 1.2g; Sodium 470mg

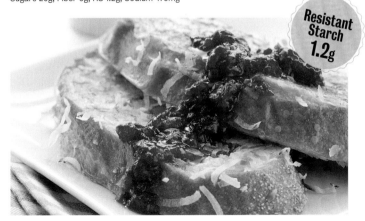

Resistant Starch 1.2g

Oatmeal-Cranberry Muffin

PREP: 5 MINUTES
COOK: 30 MINUTES
TOTAL TIME: 35 MINUTES
MAKES: 12 MUFFINS

- 1½ cup old-fashioned rolled oats
- ¾ cup all-purpose flour
- ¾ cup whole-wheat flour
- ⅓ cup sugar
- 2½ teaspoons baking powder
- 1 teaspoon ground cinnamon
- ½ teaspoon ground nutmeg
- ½ teaspoon salt
- 1 cup water
- ½ cup oil
- ½ cup applesauce
- 2 eggs
- ½ cup dried, sweetened cranberries

1. Preheat oven to 350°.
2. Spray a 12-muffin pan with cooking spray and reserve.
3. Combine oats, flours, sugar, baking powder, spices, and salt in a bowl.
4. In a separate bowl whisk water, oil, applesauce, and eggs until incorporated.
5. Combine wet and dry ingredients and add cranberries.
6. Distribute batter evenly into muffin pan. Bake until a toothpick in the center comes out clean and tops are browned, 30–35 minutes.

Serving size: 1 muffin with 1 TBSP almond butter | Calories 317; Fat 18.5g (sat 1.75g, mono 10g, poly 6g); Cholesterol 35mg; Protein 7g; Carbohydrate 33g; Sugars 11.5g; Fiber 4g; RS 1g; Sodium 241mg

Resistant
Starch
1g

Spinach & Egg Breakfast Wrap with Avocado & Pepper Jack Cheese

PREP: 10 MINUTES
COOK: 5 MINUTES
TOTAL TIME: 15 MINUTES
MAKES: 4 SERVINGS

Nonstick cooking spray
1 (5-ounce) box or bag baby spinach, chopped
4 eggs
4 egg whites
½ teaspoon salt
¼ teaspoon pepper
4 ounces shredded pepper jack cheese
1 avocado, sliced
4 whole-wheat tortillas

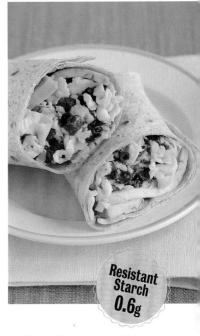

Resistant Starch
0.6g

1. Spray a nonstick skillet over medium-high heat.
2. Add spinach and cook, stirring, until wilted, 2 minutes.
3. Whisk together eggs and egg whites in a small bowl. Add eggs to skillet and cook, stirring, until cooked through, 3–4 minutes. Season with salt and pepper.
4. Place ¼ of egg mixture in the center of each tortilla, and sprinkle with 1 ounce cheese.
5. Top with 4 slices avocado and fold, burrito-style. Slice in half and serve.

Serving size: 1 wrap | Calories 366; Fat 22g (sat 8g, mono 7g, poly 2g); Cholesterol 242mg; Protein 22g; Carbohydrate 30g; Sugars 1g; Fiber 7g; RS 0.6g; Sodium 666mg

Potato-Crusted Spinach Quiche

PREP: 20 MINUTES
COOK: 1 HOUR
TOTAL TIME: 1 HOUR 20 MINUTES
MAKES: 4 SERVINGS

- 1 tablespoon olive oil, divided
- 1 (20-ounce) package refrigerated shredded potatoes (about 3½ cups)
- 1 large egg white, whisked
- 1 tablespoon all-purpose flour
- ½ teaspoon salt
- 6 ounces fresh spinach
- ¼ cup chopped onion
- 2 tablespoons water
- 6 large eggs
- ¼ cup part-skim ricotta cheese
- ¼ teaspoon freshly ground black pepper
- 2 ounces Swiss cheese, shredded (about ½ cup)
- 1 ounce Canadian bacon, finely chopped

1. Preheat oven to 400°. Coat inside of a 9-inch deep-dish pie plate with 1 teaspoon olive oil; set aside.

2. Combine potatoes and egg white in a large bowl; toss lightly. Add flour and salt; toss to coat. Transfer to pie plate, and pat evenly into bottom and sides to form crust. Drizzle remaining 2 teaspoons oil over crust. Bake for 15 minutes or until edges begin to brown. Remove from oven. Reduce oven temperature to 350°.

3. While crust bakes, place spinach, onion, and 2 tablespoons water in a microwave-safe bowl. Microwave at HIGH 2 minutes or until spinach begins to wilt; drain. Place spinach mixture in a colander, and squeeze to drain; coarsely chop, and set aside.

4. Combine eggs and ricotta in a large mixing bowl; stir until smooth. Add black pepper. Stir in spinach mixture, half of Swiss cheese, and bacon.

5. Pour egg mixture over potato crust; spread with the back of a spoon to distribute evenly, leaving a ½-inch crust along the outer edge. Sprinkle remaining Swiss cheese on top. Bake at 350° for 50–55 minutes, until puffed and golden. Cool on a wire rack 10–15 minutes before serving. Slice into 4 equal pieces and serve.

Serving size: ¼ of quiche | Calories 380; Fat 17g (sat 6g, mono 7g, poly 2g); Cholesterol 340mg; Protein 20g; Carbohydrate 37g; Sugars 1g; Fiber 6g; RS 1.4g; Sodium 720mg

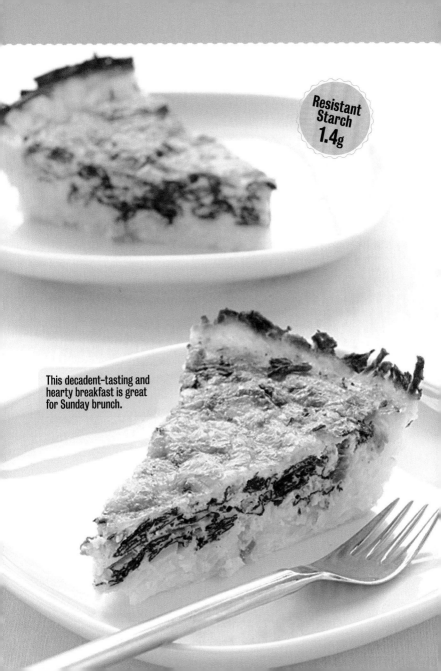

Resistant Starch 1.4g

This decadent-tasting and hearty breakfast is great for Sunday brunch.

Banana & Almond Butter Toast

PREP: 5 MINUTES
TOTAL TIME: 5 MINUTES
MAKES: 1 SERVING

> 1 tablespoon almond butter
> 1 slice rye bread, toasted
> 1 banana, sliced

1. Spread almond butter on toast.
2. Top with banana slices.

Serving size: 1 piece of toast | Calories 280; Fat 11g
(sat 1g, mono 7g, poly 2.5g); Cholesterol 0mg; Protein 6g; Carbohydrate 44g; Sugars 16g;
Fiber 5g; RS 5.6g; Sodium 260mg

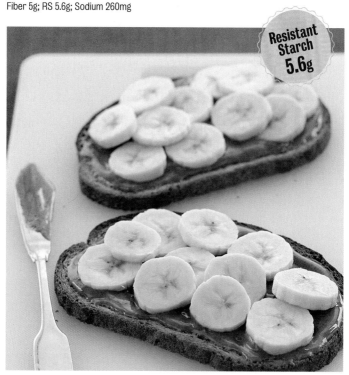

Resistant Starch 5.6g

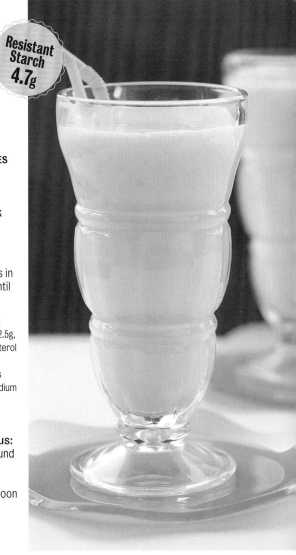

Resistant Starch 4.7g

Banana Shake

PREP: 5 MINUTES
TOTAL TIME: 5 MINUTES
MAKES: 1 SERVING

    1 banana
    1½ cups 1%
       low-fat milk
    2 teaspoons
       honey
    ½ cup ice

1. Place all ingredients in a blender; process until smooth.

Serving size: 1½ cups
Calories 300; Fat 4g (sat 2.5g, mono 1g, poly 0g); Cholesterol 20mg; Protein 14g; Carbohydrate 57g; Sugars 44g; Fiber 3g; RS 4.7g; Sodium 170mg

Variations:
■ **Banana Shake Plus:** Add 2 teaspoons ground flaxseed.
■ **Banana-Cocoa Shake:** Add 1 tablespoon unsweetened cocoa.
■ **Banana-Berry Shake:** Add ¼ cup berries (any variety).

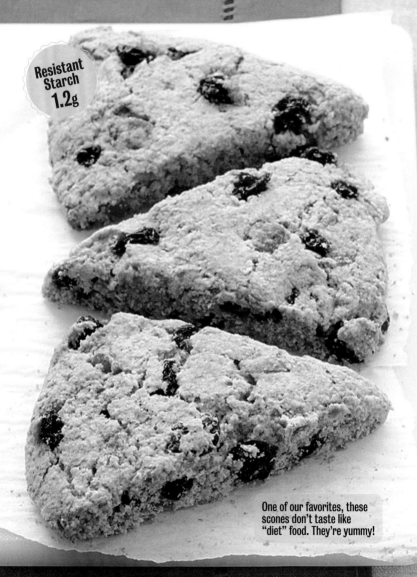

Resistant Starch 1.2g

One of our favorites, these scones don't taste like "diet" food. They're yummy!

Cherry-Ginger Scones

PREP: 20 MINUTES
BAKE: 25 MINUTES
TOTAL TIME: 45 MINUTES
MAKES: 8 SERVINGS

- 1½ cups whole-wheat pastry flour
- 1 cup old-fashioned rolled oats
- ¼ cup packed brown sugar
- 2 teaspoons baking powder
- ½ teaspoon baking soda
- ¼ teaspoon salt
- ½ cup unsalted butter
- 1 cup dried cherries
- ½ cup crystallized ginger, coarsely chopped
- ¼ cup low-fat buttermilk
- 2 large egg whites, whisked
  All-purpose flour (as needed)

1. Preheat oven to 350°. Line a baking sheet with parchment paper and set aside.
2. Combine flour, oats, brown sugar, baking powder, baking soda, and salt in a food processor. Process 10 seconds or until oats are finely chopped. Add butter; process until mixture resembles coarse meal.
3. Transfer flour mixture to a large mixing bowl; stir in cherries and crystallized ginger.
4. Combine buttermilk and egg whites in a small bowl; stir with a whisk. Add buttermilk mixture to flour mixture; stir just until a sticky dough forms.
5. Transfer dough to parchment paper–lined baking sheet, and pat into a 9-inch circle (about 1-inch thick). Sprinkle with all-purpose flour, if necessary, to keep the dough from sticking to hands. Divide the dough into 8 equal wedges. Separate wedges slightly, and bake at 350° for 25 minutes or until golden brown and a wooden pick inserted in center comes out clean.

Serving size: 1 scone | Calories 348; Fat 13g (sat 7.5g, mono 3g, poly 1g); Cholesterol 31mg; Protein 6g; Carbohydrate 53g; Sugars 20g; Fiber 5g; RS 1.2g; Sodium 271mg

Sharp Cheddar & Egg on Rye

PREP: 5 MINUTES
COOK: 5 MINUTES
TOTAL TIME: 10 MINUTES
MAKES: 1 SERVING

Cooking spray
1 large egg
2 slices rye bread, toasted
1 slice sharp Cheddar cheese
1 small apple, cored and sliced

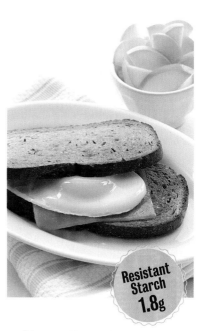

1. Heat a nonstick skillet over medium heat. Coat pan with cooking spray. Add egg; cook until set, about 3 minutes.
2. Top toast with cheese; place egg over cheese. Serve with apple slices on the side.

Resistant Starch 1.8g

Serving size: 1 sandwich and 1 apple | Calories 420; Fat 18g (sat 8g, mono 5g, poly 1.5g); Cholesterol 240mg; Protein 19g; Carbohydrate 49g; Sugars 18g; Fiber 7g; RS 1.8g; Sodium 620mg

Banana–Nut Oatmeal

PREP: 5 MINUTES
COOK: 5 MINUTES
TOTAL TIME: 10 MINUTES
MAKES: 1 SERVING

- ½ cup old–fashioned rolled oats
- 1 cup water
- 1 banana, sliced
- 1 tablespoon chopped walnuts
- 1 teaspoon cinnamon

1. Combine oats and 1 cup water in a small microwave-safe bowl. Microwave at HIGH 3 minutes.
2. Top with banana slices, walnuts, and cinnamon.

Serving size: 1½ cups | Calories 310; Fat 8g (sat 1g, mono 1.5g, poly 4.5g); Cholesterol 0mg; Protein 8g; Carbohydrate 57g; Sugars 16g; Fiber 9g; RS 5.2g; Sodium 0mg

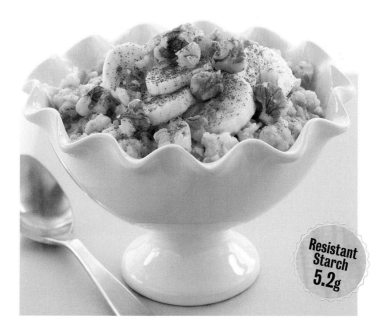

Resistant Starch 5.2g

Steel-Cut Oatmeal with Salted Caramel Topping

PREP: 5 MINUTES
COOK: 15 MINUTES
TOTAL TIME: 20 MINUTES
MAKES: 4 SERVINGS

  1 cup uncooked instant steel-cut oats
  3 cups 1 % milk
  ¼ cup light brown sugar
  ½ teaspoon salt
  ¼ cup whipped cream
  ½ cup fresh berries

1. Preheat oven to 400°.
2. Over high heat in a medium saucepan, bring oatmeal and milk to a boil. Reduce heat and simmer until oatmeal is cooked but not mushy, 7–8 minutes.
3. Remove from heat, and distribute among four 6-ounce ramekins, arranged on a rimmed baking sheet.
4. Combine sugar and salt, and sprinkle evenly on top of ramekins. Place ramekins in oven for 3–4 minutes, until sugar is melted.
5. Remove from oven, and turn oven to broil. Broil ramekins until sugar is browned and bubbly, watching carefully that they don't burn, 2–3 minutes.
6. Remove from oven, and top each oatmeal brûlée with 1 tablespoon of whipped cream and 1 tablespoon fresh berries.

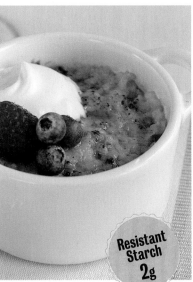

Serving size: 1 ramekin
Calories 242; Fat 6g (sat 3g, mono 2g, poly 1g); Cholesterol 20mg; Protein 9g; Carbohydrate 39g; Sugars 25g; Fiber 2g; RS 2g; Sodium 229mg

Resistant Starch
2g

Cornflakes, Low-Fat Milk & Berries

PREP: 5 MINUTES
TOTAL TIME: 5 MINUTES
MAKES: 1 SERVING

- 2 cups cornflakes
- 1 cup 1% low-fat milk
- 1 cup berries, fresh or frozen, thawed

1. Place cornflakes in a small bowl. Top with milk and berries.

Serving size: 3 cups | Calories 370; Fat 3g (sat 1.5g, mono 1g, poly 0g); Cholesterol 10mg; Protein 13g; Carbohydrate 78g; Sugars 27g; Fiber 6g; RS 1.8g; Sodium 640mg

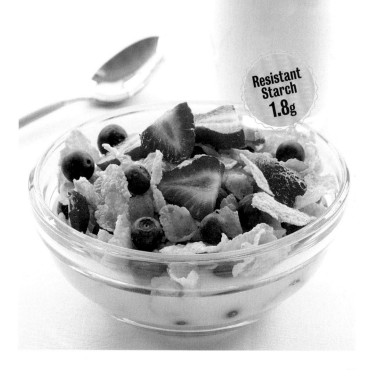

Resistant Starch 1.8g

Blueberry Oat Pancakes with Maple Yogurt

PREP: 5 MINUTES
COOK: 10 MINUTES
TOTAL TIME: 15 MINUTES
MAKES: 2 SERVINGS

    Cooking spray
1 cup old-fashioned rolled oats
½ cup low-fat cottage cheese
2 large eggs
1 teaspoon vanilla extract
1 cup blueberries
¾ cup plain low-fat Greek yogurt
1 tablespoon maple syrup

1. Combine oats, cottage cheese, eggs, and vanilla in a blender or food processor; process until smooth. Gently stir in the blueberries.
2. Heat a large nonstick skillet over medium heat. Coat pan with cooking spray. Spoon about 2 tablespoons batter per pancake into pan. Cook 3 minutes or until tops are covered with bubbles and edges look cooked. Carefully turn pancakes over, and cook 3 more minutes or until golden.
3. Combine yogurt and maple syrup; serve alongside pancakes.

Serving size: 3 (3-inch) pancakes and about ½ cup yogurt mixture
Calories 410; Fat 12g (sat 3.5g, mono 3g, poly 2g); Cholesterol 220mg; Protein 26g; Carbohydrate 50g; Sugars 20g; Fiber 6g; RS 4.6g; Sodium 330mg

These delicious, hearty pancakes are totally guilt-free!

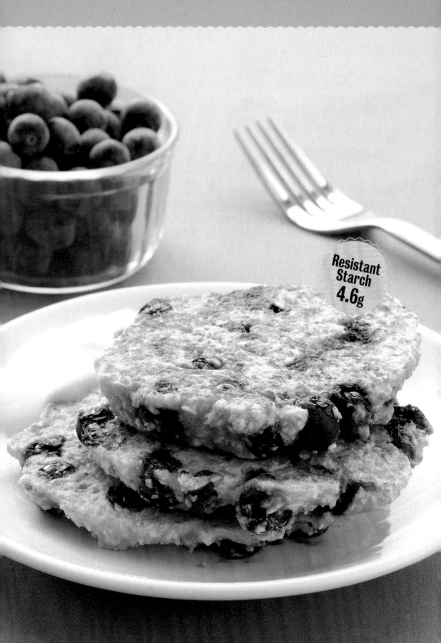

Resistant
Starch
4.6g

Resistant
Starch
4g

Three-Bean Soup with Canadian Bacon

PREP: 5 MINUTES
COOK: 25 MINUTES
TOTAL TIME: 30 MINUTES
MAKES: 4 SERVINGS

Cooking spray
1 tablespoon olive oil
1 cup diced onion
2 cloves garlic
4 cups low-sodium chicken stock
1 large zucchini, cut into small dice (about 2 cups)
1 cup drained and rinsed low-sodium cannellini beans
1 cup drained and rinsed kidney beans
1 cup drained and rinsed black beans
¼ teaspoon salt
¼ teaspoon pepper
2 slices (2 ounces) Canadian bacon, finely diced

1. Heat oil in a saucepan over medium-high heat.
2. Add onion and cook until soft, 6 minutes.
3. Add garlic and cook an additional minute.
4. Add zucchini and cook, stirring, 3–4 minutes.
5. Add stock, beans, salt, and pepper, and bring to a boil. Reduce heat, and simmer over very low heat until slightly thickened, 15 minutes.
6. While soup is simmering, spray a skillet with nonstick cooking spray, and cook bacon until crisp, 3 minutes.
7. Divide soup among 4 bowls, and top each bowl with 1 tablespoon crisped bacon.

Serving size: 2 cups soup plus 1 tablespoon crisped Canadian bacon | Calories 271; Fat 7g (sat 1g, mono 4g, poly 1g); Cholesterol 5mg; Protein 18g; Carbohydrate 38g; Sugars 6g; Fiber 11g; RS 4g; Sodium 504mg

This superfast soup is the ultimate slimming lunch. Eat it with a whole-grain roll.

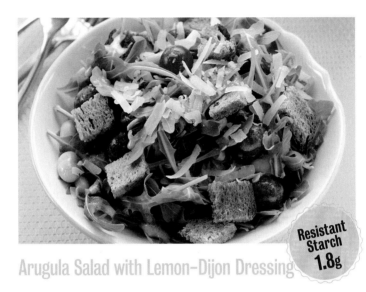

Resistant Starch 1.8g

Arugula Salad with Lemon–Dijon Dressing

PREP: 7 MINUTES
TOTAL TIME: 7 MINUTES
MAKES: 1 SERVING

  1 tablespoon lemon juice
  1 teaspoon olive oil
  1 teaspoon Dijon mustard
  3 cups arugula
  ½ cup grape tomatoes
  ½ cup canned white beans, rinsed and
      drained
  2 slices rye bread, toasted and cut into
      1-inch cubes
  1 tablespoon shredded Parmesan cheese

1. Combine first 3 ingredients (through mustard) in a small bowl, stirring with a whisk.

2. Combine arugula, tomatoes, and beans in a large bowl. Add dressing; toss gently.

3. Top with rye bread, croutons, and cheese.

Serving size: 5 cups | Calories 400; Fat 10g (sat 2g, mono 4g, poly 1.5g); Cholesterol 5mg; Protein 18g; Carbohydrate 61g; Sugars 7g; Fiber 11g; RS 1.8g; Sodium 710mg

Chicken Pita Sandwich

PREP: 5 MINUTES
TOTAL TIME: 5 MINUTES
MAKES: 1 SERVING

- 1 cup baby spinach
- ½ cup (4 ounces) cooked skinless, boneless chicken breast, sliced into ½-inch strips
- ½ cup sliced red bell pepper
- 2 tablespoons low-fat Italian vinaigrette
- 1 (6-inch) whole-grain pita, cut in half

1. Combine spinach, chicken, bell pepper, and vinaigrette in a bowl; toss gently.
2. Serve in pita halves.

Serving size: 2 stuffed pita halves | Calories 400; Fat 10g (sat 1.5g, mono 1.5g, poly 2g); Cholesterol 95mg; Protein 43g; Carbohydrate 36g; Sugars 5g; Fiber 6g; RS 1g; Sodium 670mg

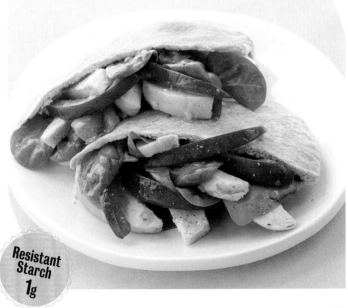

Resistant
Starch
1g

Express Lunch Plate

PREP: 5 MINUTES
TOTAL TIME: 5 MINUTES
MAKES: 1 SERVING

- 1 large hard-cooked egg
- 1 (1-ounce) Cheddar cheese wedge
- 1 apple, cored and sliced
- 3 rye crispbread crackers

1. Arrange all ingredients on a plate and enjoy.

Serving size: 1 plate | Calories 400; Fat 15g (sat 8g, mono 5g, poly 1g); Cholesterol 240mg; Protein 16g; Carbohydrate 51g; Sugars 20g; Fiber 9g; RS 1g; Sodium 320mg

Resistant Starch 1g

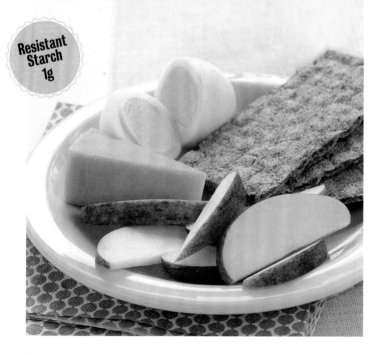

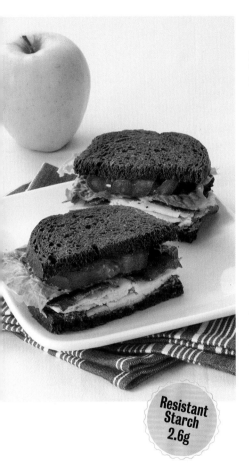

Resistant Starch 2.6g

Pesto Turkey Club

PREP: 5 MINUTES
TOTAL TIME: 5 MINUTES
MAKES: 1 SERVING

- 2 teaspoons prepared pesto
- 2 slices pumpernickel bread
- 1 (1-ounce) slice turkey
- 1 low-sodium slice turkey bacon, cooked
- 2 romaine lettuce leaves
- 4 slices tomato
- 1 apple

1. Spread pesto on 1 slice of bread. Top with turkey, turkey bacon, lettuce, tomato, and remaining bread slice. Cut sandwich in half using a sharp knife.
2. Serve sandwich with apple.

Serving size: 1 sandwich and 1 apple | Calories 390; Fat 11g (sat 3g, mono 4g, poly 1g); Cholesterol 32mg; Protein 20g; Carbohydrate 60g; Sugars 23g; Fiber 10g; RS 2.6g; Sodium 614mg

Banana-Nut Elvis Wrap

PREP: 5 MINUTES
TOTAL TIME: 5 MINUTES
MAKES: 4 SERVINGS

  4 (6-inch) whole-wheat wraps
  ½ cup chunky natural-style peanut butter
  2 large bananas, sliced
  2 tablespoons honey

1. Spread 2 tablespoons peanut butter on bottom third of each wrap, leaving 2-inch border on each side.
2. Top each wrap with ½ sliced banana and about 2 teaspoons honey.
3. Roll up wrap, slice in half, and serve immediately.

Serving size: 1 wrap | Calories 354; Fat 17g (sat 3g, mono 8g, poly 5g); Cholesterol 0mg; Protein 11g; Carbohydrate 51g; Sugars 20g; Fiber 6g; RS 3g; Sodium 328mg

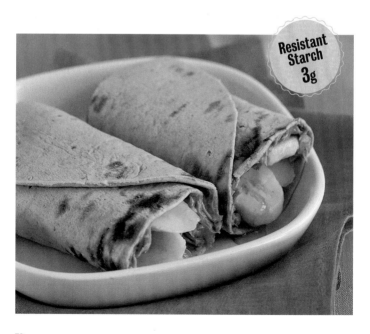

Resistant Starch 3g

Grilled Cheese & Tomato on Rye

PREP: 5 MINUTES
COOK: 6 MINUTES
TOTAL TIME: 11 MINUTES
MAKES: 4 SERVINGS

Cooking spray
8 slices rye bread
4 tablespoons grainy mustard
8 ounces reduced-fat Cheddar cheese, sliced
1 beefsteak tomato, sliced

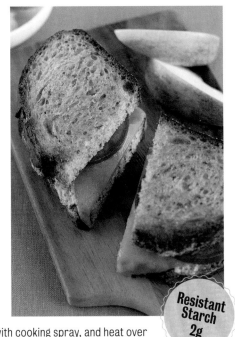

Resistant Starch 2g

1. Spray a nonstick pan with cooking spray, and heat over medium-high heat.
2. Spread 1 tablespoon mustard on each of 4 slices of bread, then top each with 2 slices of cheese and 1 slice of tomato. Top with an additional slice of bread.
3. Place sandwiches in pan, and place another pan on top of the sandwiches.
4. Cook until bottoms of sandwiches are browned, 2–3 minutes. Flip and continue cooking an additional 2–3 minutes, until bread is golden and cheese is melted.

Serving size: 1 sandwich | Calories 355; Fat 14g (sat 7g, mono 4g, poly 1g); Cholesterol 32mg; Protein 22g; Carbohydrate 35g; Sugars 4g; Fiber 5g; RS 2g; Sodium 1,192mg

Roast Beef Pumpernickel Sandwich with Roasted Red Pepper, Arugula & Goat Cheese

PREP: 10 MINUTES
TOTAL TIME: 10 MINUTES
MAKES: 4 SERVINGS

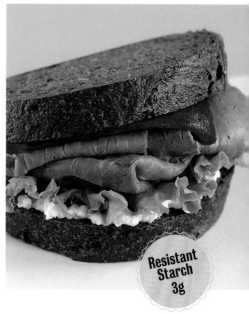

Resistant Starch 3g

3 ounces goat cheese, softened

8 slices pumpernickel bread

4 green lettuce leaves

12 ounces thinly sliced lean roast beef

4 jarred roasted red peppers (2 ounces each), drained, rinsed, patted dry, and halved

4 teaspoons balsamic vinegar

1. Spread the goat cheese on 4 slices of the bread.
2. Arrange 1 lettuce leaf on each of the 4 cheese-topped bread slices, then layer each with 3 ounces roast beef.
3. Top with red peppers, drizzle with balsamic vinegar, and cover with second slice of bread. Serve.

Serving size: 1 sandwich | Calories 380; Fat 11g (sat 5g, mono 4g, poly 1g); Cholesterol 74mg; Protein 33g; Carbohydrate 38g; Sugars 3g; Fiber 4g; RS 3g; Sodium 653mg

Lunch Shake

PREP: 5 MINUTES
TOTAL TIME: 5 MINUTES
MAKES: 2 SERVINGS

- 1 cup fresh or frozen raspberries
- 1 cup shredded kale
- 1 cup ice
- ¾ cup fat-free plain yogurt
- ½ banana
- 2 tablespoons honey
- 1 tablespoon natural almond butter
- 1 tablespoon wheat germ

1. Combine all ingredients in a blender, and blend until smooth. Serve immediately.

Serving size: 8 ounces
Calories 239; Fat 6g (sat 1g, mono 3g, poly 2g); Cholesterol 2mg; Protein 8g; Carbohydrate 45g; Sugars 29g; Fiber 6g; RS 1g; Sodium 102mg

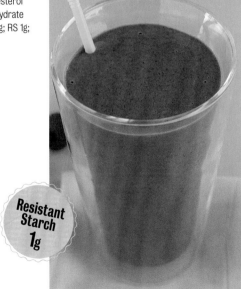

Resistant Starch 1g

Red Grape & Tuna Salad Pita

PREP: 7 MINUTES
TOTAL TIME: 7 MINUTES
MAKES: 1 SERVING

- ½ can (3 ounces) tuna in water, drained
- ½ cup red grapes, halved
- 1 tablespoon slivered almonds
- 1 tablespoon chopped fresh mint
- 1 tablespoon lemon juice
- 2 teaspoons olive oil
- ⅛ teaspoon black pepper
- 1 whole-grain pita, halved

1. Combine first 7 ingredients (through pepper) in a small bowl. Toss gently. Serve in pita halves.

Serving size: 2 stuffed pita halves | Calories 410; Fat 15g
(sat 1.5g, mono 9g, poly 3g); Cholesterol 45mg; Protein 28g; Carbohydrate 45g; Sugars 14g; Fiber 6g; RS 1g; Sodium 700mg

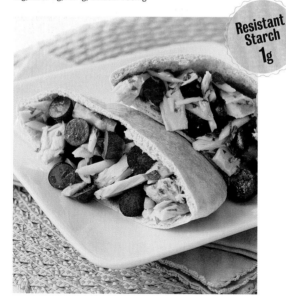

Resistant Starch 1g

Black Bean & Zucchini Quesadillas

PREP: 5 MINUTES
COOK: 2 MINUTES
TOTAL TIME: 7 MINUTES
MAKES: 1 SERVING

- ½ cup canned black beans, rinsed and drained
- 2 tablespoons salsa
- ½ cup finely chopped zucchini
- 4 (6-inch) corn tortillas
- 4 tablespoons shredded Cheddar cheese

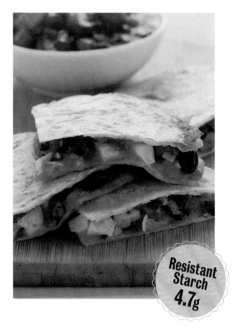

Resistant Starch 4.7g

1. Combine beans and salsa in a small bowl; mash with a fork. Stir in zucchini.
2. Layer 2 tortillas with half of the bean mixture, sprinkle with 2 tablespoons cheese, and top with remaining 2 tortillas. Repeat with remaining tortillas, bean mixture, and cheese.
3. In toaster oven, cook 1 minute per side, until cheese is melted.

Serving size: 2 quesadillas | Calories 400; Fat 11g (sat 6g, mono 0.5g, poly 1.5g); Cholesterol 30mg; Protein 18g; Carbohydrate 65g; Sugars 4g; Fiber 13g; RS 4.7g; Sodium 670mg

Curried Egg Salad Sandwich

PREP: 7 MINUTES
TOTAL TIME: 7 MINUTES
MAKES: 1 SERVING

- 2 hard-cooked eggs, chopped
- 2 tablespoons plain low-fat Greek yogurt
- 2 tablespoons chopped red bell pepper
- ¼ teaspoon curry powder
- Dash of salt
- ⅛ teaspoon pepper
- 2 slices rye bread, toasted
- ½ cup fresh spinach
- 1 orange, sliced

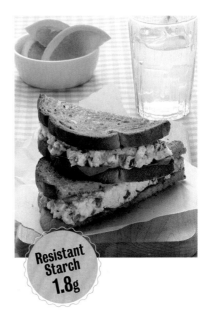

Resistant Starch
1.8g

1. Combine eggs, yogurt, bell pepper, curry powder, salt, and pepper in a small bowl; stir well.
2. Place spinach on 1 slice of bread, and top with egg salad. Place other piece of bread on top. Slice in half on the diagonal with a sharp knife. Serve with orange slices.

Serving size: 1 sandwich and 1 orange | Calories 414; Fat 14g (sat 4g, mono 5g, poly 2g); Cholesterol 426mg; Protein 22g; Carbohydrate 51g; Sugars 18g; Fiber 8g; RS 1.8g; Sodium 654mg

Big Chopped Salad

PREP: 5 MINUTES
TOTAL TIME: 5 MINUTES
MAKES: 1 SERVING

- 3 cups mixed salad greens
- ½ cup canned no-salt-added garbanzo beans, rinsed and drained
- ½ cup shredded carrots
- ½ cup shredded red cabbage
- 1 tablespoon grated Parmesan cheese
- 2 tablespoons chopped walnuts
- 2 tablespoons dried cranberries
- 2 tablespoons low-fat balsamic vinaigrette

1. Combine first 7 ingredients (through cranberries) in a large bowl.
2. Toss with vinaigrette and serve.

Serving size: 4½ cups | Calories 390; Fat 14g (sat 2g, mono 2g, poly 8g); Cholesterol 5mg; Protein 15g; Carbohydrate 60g; Sugars 23g; Fiber 13g; RS 2.1g; Sodium 630mg

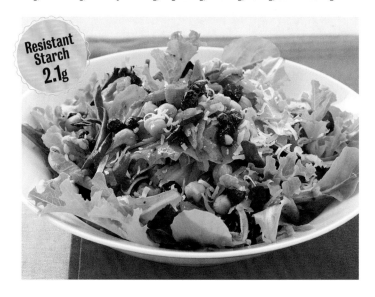

Resistant Starch
2.1g

Ham, Pear & Swiss Cheese Sandwich

PREP: 10 MINUTES
TOTAL TIME: 10 MINUTES
MAKES: 1 SERVING

- 1 tablespoon plain low-fat Greek yogurt
- ¼ teaspoon dried dill
- 2 slices pumpernickel bread
- 1 (1-ounce) slice lean ham
- 1 small pear, thinly sliced
- 1 (1-ounce) slice low-sodium Swiss cheese

1. Combine yogurt and dill in a small bowl; stir until blended.
2. Spread yogurt mixture on 1 slice of bread. Top with ham, half of the pear slices, cheese, and remaining bread slice. Slice in half using a sharp knife. Serve with remaining pear slices on the side.

Serving size: 1 sandwich and 1 pear | Calories 410; Fat 13g (sat 6g, mono 4g, poly 1g); Cholesterol 43mg; Protein 22g; Carbohydrate 55g; Sugars 16g; Fiber 9g; RS 2.6g; Sodium 710mg

Resistant Starch
2.6g

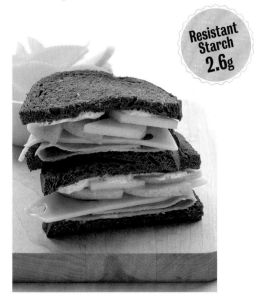

Black Bean, Avocado, Brown Rice & Chicken Wrap

PREP: 15 MINUTES
TOTAL TIME: 15 MINUTES
MAKES: 4 SERVINGS

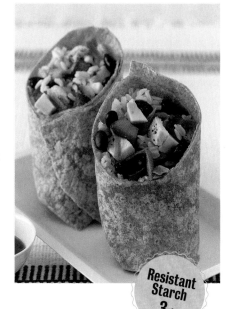

Resistant Starch 3g

- ½ teaspoon salt
- ¼ teaspoon black pepper
- 1⅓ cup low-sodium black beans, drained and rinsed
- 1 teaspoon chili powder
- ½ teaspoon cumin
- ¼ teaspoon chili flakes
- 4 (10-inch) whole-wheat wraps
- 1⅓ cups cooked brown rice
- 8 ounces grilled chicken breast, sliced
- 1 small carrot, shredded (about 1 cup)
- ½ avocado, pitted and diced
- 1 Roma tomato, seeded and chopped (½ cup)
- Hot sauce for serving, optional

1. Combine first 6 ingredients in a small bowl and toss.
2. Place one wrap on a clean work surface. Spoon ⅓ cup rice onto bottom of wrap. Add ⅓ cup bean mixture, 2 ounces chicken, and ¼ cup shredded carrot, then top with 1 tablespoon avocado and 2 tablespoons tomato.
3. Seal wrap, slice in half, and serve immediately with hot sauce on the side, if desired.

Serving size: 1 wrap | Calories 425; Fat 9g (sat 1g, mono 3g, poly 1g); Cholesterol 48mg; Protein 31g; Carbohydrate 60g; Sugars 7g; Fiber 12g; RS 3g; Sodium 636mg

CarbLovers Club Sandwich

PREP: 15 MINUTES
COOK: 10 MINUTES
TOTAL TIME: 25 MINUTES
MAKES: 4 SERVINGS

- ¾ cup drained and rinsed low-sodium cannellini beans from a 15-ounce can
- 2 cloves roasted garlic (such as Christopher Ranch brand)
- 1 tablespoon olive oil
- ¼ teaspoon salt
- ¼ teaspoon pepper
- 12 slices thin whole-wheat bread, toasted
- 8 leaves butter lettuce
- 1 beefsteak tomato, sliced
- 1 avocado, pitted and sliced
- 8 slices turkey bacon, cooked according to directions and drained

1. Mash beans, garlic, olive oil, salt, and pepper with a fork and reserve.
2. Arrange 4 slices bread on a work surface. Spread 3 tablespoons white-bean mixture on each slice of bread.
3. Top with 2 slices lettuce and 2 tomato slices.
4. Layer another slice of bread on each sandwich, and top each with 4 slices avocado and 2 slices turkey bacon. Top with last piece of bread.
5. Slice sandwiches in half diagonally, and secure with toothpicks.

Serving size: 1 sandwich | Calories 412; Fat 18g (sat 2g, mono 10g, poly 4g); Cholesterol 14mg; Protein 16g; Carbohydrate 47g; Sugars 5g; Fiber 12g; RS 2g; Sodium 572mg

Take a bite out of the perfect combination of creamy avocado, salty bacon, and cool tomato.

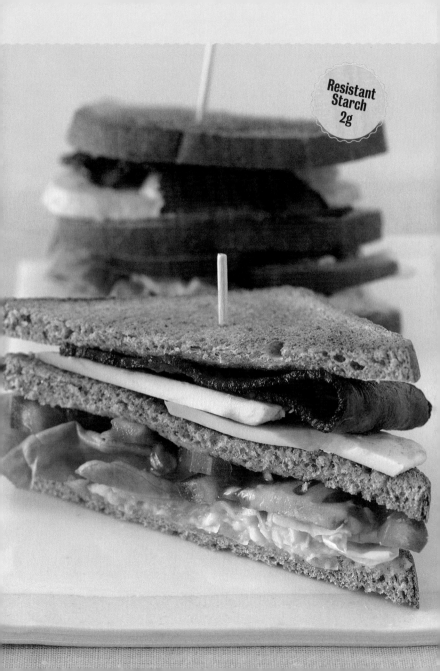

Resistant
Starch
2g

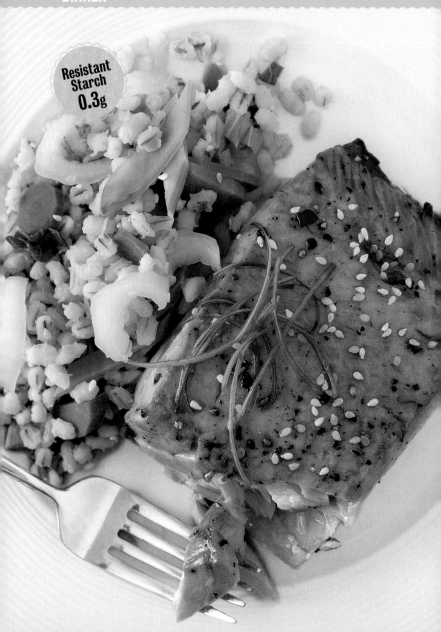

Resistant
Starch
0.3g

Honey & Sesame-Glazed Salmon
with Confetti Barley Salad

PREP: 10 MINUTES
COOK: 30 MINUTES
TOTAL TIME: 40 MINUTES
MAKES: 4 SERVINGS

- ¾ cup pearled barley
- 1 (16-ounce) bag frozen stir-fry vegetables, defrosted and chopped
- 1 tablespoon toasted sesame seeds, divided
- 4 (4-ounce) skinless salmon fillets
- 3 tablespoons honey
- ¼ cup low-sodium soy sauce
- 1½ teaspoon toasted sesame oil
- ¼ teaspoon chili flakes
- ¼ cup chopped scallions

1. Preheat oven to 400°.
2. Bring a large pot of salted water to a boil.
3. Add barley, return to a boil, and boil until tender, 30 minutes. Add vegetable medley during last 3 minutes of cooking. Drain, cool slightly, and toss with 2 teaspoons sesame seeds and reserve.
4. While barley is cooking, make salmon: Combine honey, soy sauce, sesame oil, and chili flakes. Reserve 4 tablespoons of mixture. Place salmon on a baking sheet, and brush with honey-soy mixture. Bake until salmon is flaky, 15 minutes. Place reserved sauce in a small saucepan over low heat, and keep warm.
5. Divide barley mixture among 4 plates, top with a salmon fillet and 1 tablespoon warmed sauce, and sprinkle with scallions and remaining sesame seeds.

Serving size: 1 cup barley-vegetable mixture, 4 ounces salmon, and 1 tablespoon additional sauce | Calories 435; Fat 7g (sat 0g, mono 2g, poly 3g); Cholesterol 72mg; Protein 33g; Carbohydrate 53g; Sugars 16g; Fiber 9g; RS 0.3g; Sodium 615mg

> This is truly a power meal! Omega-3-packed salmon helps boost your metabolism.

Hearty Chicken Posole Stew

PREP: 10 MINUTES
COOK: 30 MINUTES
TOTAL TIME: 40 MINUTES
MAKES: 4 SERVINGS

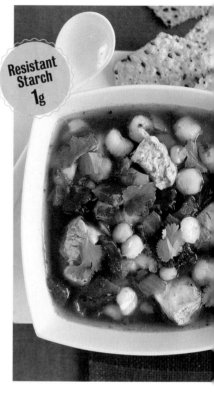

Resistant Starch 1g

- 1 tablespoon olive oil
- 1 small onion, chopped
- 2 cloves minced garlic
- 1 pound skinless, boneless chicken breast, cubed
- ¾ teaspoon cumin
- ½ teaspoon dried oregano
- 4 cups low-sodium chicken broth
- 1 (15-ounce) can fire-roasted tomatoes
- 1 (15-ounce) can hominy, rinsed and drained
- 1 tablespoon diced green chiles
- ½ teaspoon salt
- ¼ teaspoon pepper
  Fresh cilantro for garnish

1. Heat oil in a 3-quart saucepan over medium heat.
2. Add onions and cook until soft, 6–7 minutes.
3. Add garlic and cook, stirring, an additional 2 minutes.
4. Add chicken, cumin, and oregano, and cook, stirring, until just cooked through, 5 minutes.
5. Add broth, tomatoes, hominy, green chile, salt, and pepper, and bring to a boil. Reduce heat, skimming foam from top of soup, and simmer 10 minutes, until liquid has thickened slightly.
6. Divide among 4 bowls, and serve immediately with tortilla chips alongside, if desired.

Serving size: 2 cups stew | Calories 303; Fat 9g (sat 2g, mono 4g, poly 2g); Cholesterol 63mg; Protein 30g; Carbohydrate 26g; Sugars 6g; Fiber 4g; RS 1g; Sodium 743mg

Grilled Burger & Three-Bean Salad

PREP: 5 MINUTES
COOK: 15 MINUTES
TOTAL TIME: 20 MINUTES
MAKES: 2 SERVINGS

- 6 ounces lean ground sirloin or bison
- 1 teaspoon olive oil
- ½ cup green beans, fresh or frozen, thawed
- ½ cup canned white beans, rinsed and drained
- ½ cup canned kidney beans, rinsed and drained
- ½ cup carrot, peeled and chopped
- ½ cup chopped green bell pepper
- 2 (1½-ounce) whole-grain hamburger buns
- 2 tablespoons low-fat Italian vinaigrette
  Romaine lettuce leaves
- 4 tomato slices

1. Divide beef into 2 equal portions, shaping each into a ½-inch-thick patty.
2. Heat oil in a nonstick skillet over medium heat. Place patties in pan; cook 6 minutes each side or until a meat thermometer inserted into middle of burger reads 160°.
3. Combine green beans, white beans, kidney beans, carrot, bell pepper, and vinaigrette in a bowl; toss gently.
4. On the bottom of each bun, place a few lettuce leaves and 2 slices tomato; top with burger and other half of bun. Serve bean salad alongside burgers.

Serving size: 1 burger and 1 cup salad | Calories 400; Fat 11g (sat 2g, mono 4g, poly 2g); Cholesterol 45mg; Protein 29g; Carbohydrate 50g; Sugars 9g; Fiber 12g; RS 2.3g; Sodium 580mg

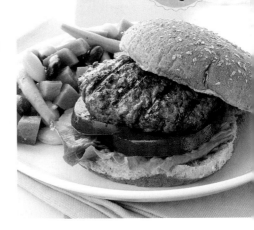

Resistant Starch 2.3g

Shrimp Stir-Fry with Ginger

PREP: 5 MINUTES
COOK: 10 MINUTES
TOTAL TIME: 15 MINUTES
MAKES: 2 SERVINGS

- 2 teaspoons dark sesame oil
- 2 tablespoons low-sodium soy sauce
- 1 tablespoon honey
- 1 tablespoon grated, peeled fresh ginger
- 2 garlic cloves, minced
- 4 cups frozen stir-fry vegetables, thawed
- 3 ounces (about 14 medium) frozen precooked shrimp, thawed
- 1½ cups cooked brown rice
- 2 tablespoons sliced almonds
- 1 scallion, chopped

1. Heat oil in a large nonstick skillet over medium heat. Add soy sauce, honey, ginger, and garlic; cook 1 minute.
2. Add vegetables, shrimp, and cooked rice; cook 8 minutes.
3. Remove from heat. Top with almonds and scallions, and serve.

Serving size: 3 cups | Calories 410; Fat 9g (sat 1.5g, mono 4g, poly 3.5g); Cholesterol 65mg; Protein 17g; Carbohydrate 61g; Sugars 14g; Fiber 6g; RS 2.6g; Sodium 710mg

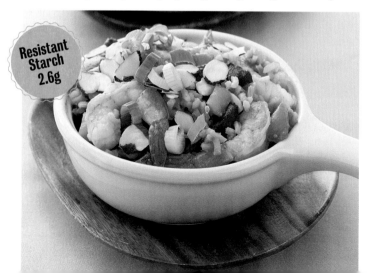

Resistant Starch 2.6g

Gnocchi with Walnut–Arugula Pesto

PREP: 5 MINUTES
COOK: 5 MINUTES
TOTAL TIME: 10 MINUTES
MAKES: 4 SERVINGS

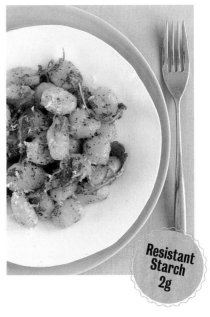

- 6 cups loosely packed arugula, divided
- 1¼ cups (1 ½ ounces) freshly grated Parmesan cheese, divided
- ¼ cup walnuts
- ½ teaspoon salt
- ¼ teaspoon ground pepper
- 2 tablespoons olive oil
- 1 tablespoon water
- 1 (14-ounce) package frozen, store-bought potato gnocchi

Resistant Starch 2g

1. Place 4 cups arugula, 1 cup Parmesan cheese, walnuts, salt, and pepper in a food processor, and pulse until incorporated, 30 seconds. With motor running, drizzle in olive oil and water, and process until smooth, another 30 seconds, adding more water by the tablespoonful if necessary.
2. Cook gnocchi according to package directions; drain. Return gnocchi to pot, and add pesto.
3. Divide remaining 2 cups arugula among 4 bowls, and toss with the gnocchi. Sprinkle with remaining Parmesan, and serve immediately.

Serving size: 2 cups gnocchi-arugula mixture | Calories 358; Fat 25g (sat 10g, mono 10g, poly 4g); Cholesterol 41mg; Protein 14g; Carbohydrate 21g; Sugars 1g; Fiber 2g; RS 2g; Sodium 605mg

Spaghetti & Turkey Meatballs in Tomato Sauce

PREP: 15 MINUTES
COOK: 30 MINUTES
TOTAL TIME: 45 MINUTES
MAKES: 5 SERVINGS

- 1 pound ground lean turkey meat
- ¾ cup finely grated Parmigiano-Reggiano cheese, divided
- ¼ cup chopped parsley, plus more for garnish
- ¼ cup fresh whole-wheat breadcrumbs (from 1 slice whole-wheat bread)
- 1 egg, beaten
- ¾ teaspoon salt, divided
- ½ teaspoon pepper, divided
- 1 tablespoon olive oil
- 1 small onion, minced (1 cup)
- 2 cloves minced garlic
- 1 (26-ounce) can low-sodium crushed tomatoes
- 1 cup canned pinto beans, rinsed and drained
- ½ pound whole-wheat spaghetti, cooked according to package directions and kept warm

1. Combine turkey, ½ cup cheese, parsley, breadcrumbs, egg, ½ teaspoon salt, and ¼ teaspoon pepper in a bowl, and form into 15 meatballs. Place meatballs on a plate and reserve.
2. Heat oil in a large saucepan over medium-high heat. Add onion, and cook until soft, 5 minutes. Add garlic, and cook an additional 2 minutes.
3. Add tomatoes, beans, and remaining salt and pepper; bring to a boil.
4. Add meatballs; return to a boil. Reduce heat, and simmer on low heat until meatballs are cooked through and sauce has thickened, 15 minutes.
5. Divide spaghetti among 5 bowls, then divide meatballs and sauce among bowls. Garnish with additional parsley and remaining ¼ cup cheese.

Serving size: 1 cup pasta, 3 meatballs, and about 1 cup sauce | Calories 439; Fat 12g (sat 3g, mono 3g, poly 1g); Cholesterol 98mg; Protein 33g; Carbohydrate 55g; Sugars 2g; Fiber 9g; RS 2g; Sodium 623mg

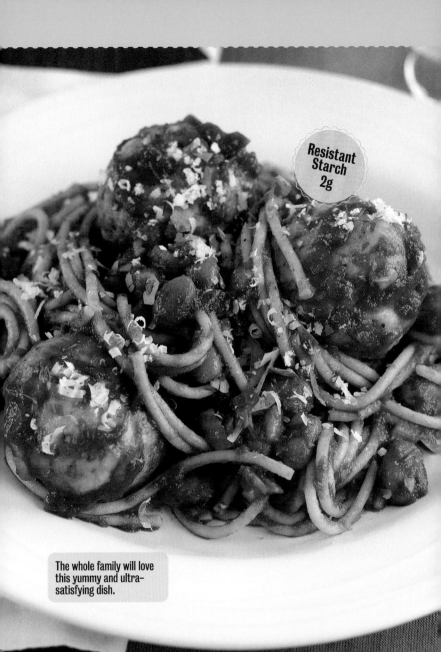

Resistant Starch 2g

The whole family will love this yummy and ultra-satisfying dish.

Pizza with Prosciutto, Tomatoes & Parmesan Cheese

PREP: 5 MINUTES
COOK: 15 MINUTES
TOTAL TIME: 20 MINUTES
MAKES: 4 SERVINGS

- 1 (12-inch) pre-baked whole-wheat pizza crust
- ¾ cup marinara sauce
- ½ cup shredded, part-skim mozzarella cheese
- ¼ cup freshly grated Parmesan cheese
- 2 thin slices (1 ounce) prosciutto di Parma
- 3 small tomatoes, sliced (4 ounces)
- 8 fresh basil leaves

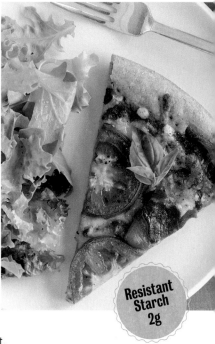

Resistant Starch 2g

1. Preheat oven to 400°.
2. Place pizza crust on a baking sheet.
3. Spread sauce evenly over crust, leaving a 1-inch border around the edges.
4. Combine cheeses, and sprinkle evenly over sauce. Top with prosciutto slices and tomatoes.
5. Bake until cheese is bubbly and crust is browned around the edges, 12–15 minutes. Remove from oven, and distribute basil leaves evenly over pizza. Let pizza set for 5 minutes. Slice into 8 pieces, and serve immediately.

Serving size: 2 slices | Calories 279; Fat 9g (sat 4g, mono 3g, poly 0g); Cholesterol 17mg; Protein 16g; Carbohydrate 38g; Sugars 6g; Fiber 7g; RS 2g; Sodium 728mg

Chicken Pasta Primavera

PREP: 5 MINUTES
COOK: 15 MINUTES
TOTAL TIME: 20 MINUTES
MAKES: 2 SERVINGS

- 4 ounces uncooked whole-grain rotini
- 2 teaspoons olive oil
- ½ cup (4 ounces) cooked skinless, boneless chicken breast, sliced into ½-inch strips
- 1 onion, vertically sliced
- 3 garlic cloves, minced
- 1 teaspoon dried oregano
- ⅛ teaspoon salt
- ⅛ teaspoon pepper
- 2 cups chopped tomato
- 1 zucchini, sliced lengthwise into ribbons
- 2 tablespoons grated Parmesan cheese

1. Cook pasta according to package directions, omitting salt and fat. Drain.
2. Meanwhile, heat oil in a nonstick skillet over medium heat. Add chicken; cook 5 minutes.
3. Add onion, garlic, oregano, salt, pepper, and tomato to pan; cook 8–10 minutes.
4. Combine chicken mixture, pasta, and zucchini ribbons; toss gently. Top with Parmesan cheese.

Serving size: 3½ cups pasta mixture | Calories 410; Fat 9g (sat 2g, mono 3.5g, poly 1g); Cholesterol 40mg; Protein 28g; Carbohydrate 61g; Sugars 13g; Fiber 12g; RS 2g; Sodium 480mg

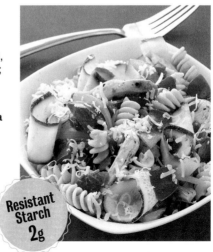

Resistant Starch 2g

Pasta with Peas, Ham & Parmesan Cheese

PREP: 5 MINUTES
COOK: 15 MINUTES
TOTAL TIME: 20 MINUTES
MAKES: 4 SERVINGS

- ½ cup light sour cream
- 1 (10-ounce) box frozen peas, defrosted
- 8 ounces uncooked whole-wheat orecchiette or bow-tie pasta
- 4 ounces lean, boneless ham, thinly sliced
- 1 cup finely grated Parmesan cheese, divided
- 2 tablespoons chopped fresh tarragon, plus more for garnish
- ½ teaspoon salt
- ½ teaspoon pepper

1. Combine sour cream and peas in a small bowl.
2. Cook the pasta according to package directions. Drain, reserving ¼ cup of the pasta water.
3. Return pasta to pot, and fold in sour cream mixture, ham, ¾ cup cheese, tarragon, salt, and pepper.

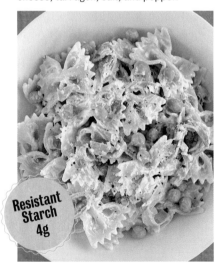

4. Divide among 4 bowls, and garnish with additional tarragon and remaining Parmesan cheese.

Serving size: 2 cups pasta

Calories 434; Fat 13g (sat 7g, mono 4g, poly 1g); Cholesterol 55mg; Protein 29g; Carbohydrate 54g; Sugars 5g; Fiber 8g; RS 4g; Sodium 538mg

Resistant Starch 4g

Black Bean Tacos

PREP: 5 MINUTES
COOK: 5 MINUTES
TOTAL TIME: 10 MINUTES
MAKES: 2 SERVINGS

- 1 (15-ounce) can no-salt-added black beans, rinsed and drained
- 6 (6-inch) corn tortillas
- 6 tablespoons shredded Cheddar cheese
- 2 cups shredded romaine lettuce
- 1 cup grated carrots
- ¼ cup salsa

1. Microwave beans on HIGH 2 minutes or until heated through.
2. Heat a nonstick skillet over medium heat. Add tortillas, one at a time; cook 1 minute on each side.
3. Divide beans evenly among tortillas. Top with even amounts of cheese, lettuce, carrot, and salsa. Fold in half and serve.

Serving size: 3 tacos
Calories 420; Fat 8g (sat 5g, mono 0.5g,poly 1g); Cholesterol 25mg; Protein 18g; Carbohydrate 69g; Sugars 5g; Fiber 17g; RS 4.7g; Sodium 420mg

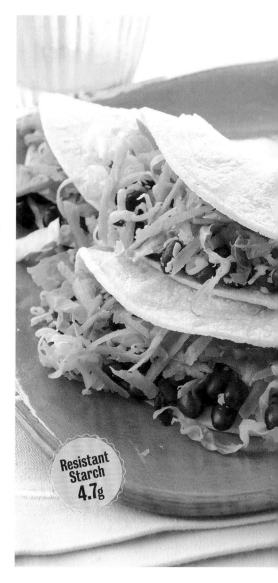

Resistant Starch 4.7g

Roasted Pork Tenderloin with Apricot-Barley Pilaf

PREP: 10 MINUTES
COOK: 30 MINUTES
TOTAL TIME: 40 MINUTES
MAKES: 4 SERVINGS

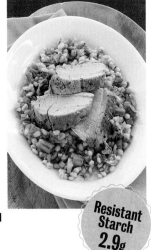

Resistant Starch 2.9g

- 1 pound pork tenderloin, trimmed of visible fat
- 1 teaspoon olive oil
- ¼ teaspoon salt
  Freshly ground black pepper
- 2 tablespoons apricot jam
- 1 tablespoon low-sodium soy sauce
- ¼ cup pecans, coarsely chopped
- 1 celery stalk, finely chopped
- 1 carrot, peeled and diced
- ¼ cup finely chopped onion
- ¾ cup water
- 3 cups quick-cooking barley, cooked
- ½ cup dried apricot halves, chopped
- ¼ cup chopped fresh parsley

1. Preheat oven to 375°.
2. Rub pork with oil; sprinkle with salt and pepper, and set aside. Combine jam and soy sauce in a small bowl; set aside.
3. Heat a large ovenproof nonstick skillet over medium-high heat. Add pecans, and toss frequently, 3–5 minutes or until fragrant. Reserve.
4. Return pan to heat; add pork. Cook 5 minutes, turning to brown on all sides. Add jam mixture, celery, carrot, and onion to pan; stir until vegetables and pork are evenly coated with sauce. Stir in the water. Bake 18–20 minutes or until a meat thermometer registers 160°.
5. Remove from oven; transfer pork to plate. Cover with foil; let stand 5 minutes.
6. Stir barley, apricots, pecans, and parsley into vegetable mixture. Slice pork into 12 pieces. Serve 3 slices pork on top of barley pilaf.

Serving size: 3 pieces pork and 1 cup pilaf | Calories 400; Fat 9g (sat 1.5g, mono 4g, poly 2g); Cholesterol 75mg; Protein 28g; Carbohydrate 54g; Sugars 15g; Fiber 7g; RS 2.9g; Sodium 390mg

Orecchiette with White Beans & Pesto

PREP: 10 MINUTES
COOK: 15 MINUTES
TOTAL TIME: 25 MINUTES
MAKES: 4 SERVINGS

- 8 ounces uncooked orecchiette or seashell pasta
- 1 teaspoon olive oil
- 2 cloves minced garlic
- 1 (15-ounce) can white kidney beans, rinsed and drained
- 3 plum tomatoes, chopped (about 1½ cups)
- ⅓ cup prepared pesto
- ¼ cup shredded Parmesan cheese

1. Cook pasta according to package directions, omitting salt and fat.
2. While the pasta cooks, heat olive oil and garlic in a large nonstick skillet over medium-high heat until garlic is fragrant. Add beans and tomato; reduce heat to low, and cook, stirring occasionally, about 5–7 minutes.
3. Drain pasta, and add to bean mixture. Add pesto; toss to combine. Divide evenly among 4 servings dishes. Top each serving with 1 tablespoon Parmesan cheese.

Serving size: 1¼ cups pasta mixture | Calories 420; Fat 11g (sat 2.5g, mono 4g, poly 5g); Cholesterol 5mg; Protein 18g; Carbohydrate 63g; Sugars 5g; Fiber 7g; RS 4.4g; Sodium 360mg

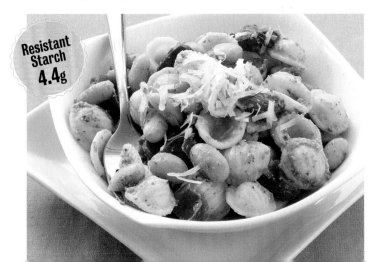

Resistant Starch 4.4g

Resistant
Starch
0.2g

Bison Sliders with Guacamole

PREP: 20 MINUTES
COOK: 5 MINUTES
TOTAL TIME: 25 MINUTES
MAKES: 4 SERVINGS

- 1 large avocado
- 1 tablespoon reduced-fat sour cream
  Juice and zest of 1 lime
- 1 tablespoon finely chopped jalapeño pepper
- 2 tablespoons chopped cilantro
- ¾ teaspoon salt, divided
- ½ teaspoon pepper, divided
- 1 pound ground bison
- 1 clove minced garlic
- 1 small head butter lettuce, inner leaves separated
- 8 whole-wheat slider buns
- 2 Roma tomatoes, thinly sliced
- ½ small red onion, sliced into rings

1. In a medium bowl, mash avocado, sour cream, lime juice and zest, jalapeño, cilantro, ½ teaspoon salt, and ¼ teaspoon pepper until chunky. Press plastic wrap onto surface of guacamole, and refrigerate.
2. Combine bison, garlic, and remaining salt and pepper in a small bowl. Form into 8 2-ounce patties, transfer to a plate, and set aside.
3. Preheat a grill or grill pan over medium-high heat. Grill sliders until thoroughly cooked; 4 minutes per side for medium.
4. Layer one lettuce leaf, a slice of tomato, and an onion ring on bottom half of each bun, and top with 2 tablespoons guacamole. Add a slider, and top with other half of bun.

Serving size: 2 sliders | Calories 444; Fat 24g (sat 8g, mono 11g, poly 3g); Cholesterol 61mg; Protein 23g; Carbohydrate 38g; Sugars 7g; Fiber 9g; RS 0.2g; Sodium 544mg

These juicy sliders are killer! Make them for a party or an easy weeknight dinner.

Sausage, Tomato, White Bean & Corkscrew Pasta Toss

PREP: 5 MINUTES
COOK: 20 MINUTES
TOTAL TIME: 25 MINUTES
MAKES: 4 SERVINGS

- 1 tablespoon olive oil
- 2 links (6 ounces) low-fat Italian sausage, thinly sliced
- 1 (26-ounce) can diced tomatoes, juice included
- 1 (15-ounce) can unsalted cannellini beans, rinsed and drained
- 2 teaspoons dried oregano or 1 teaspoon fresh
- ½ teaspoon chili flakes
- ½ pound whole-wheat fusilli pasta, cooked according to package directions
- ¼ cup freshly grated Parmesan cheese
- 2 tablespoons chopped parsley

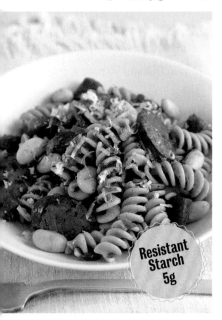

1. Heat oil in a sauté pan over medium-high heat.
2. Add sausage, and cook until browned, 5–6 minutes.
3. Add tomatoes with juices, beans, oregano, chili flakes, salt, and pepper, and bring to a low boil.
4. Reduce heat, and cook until liquid reduces slightly, 3–4 minutes.
5. Stir in pasta, and heat through, 2–3 minutes.
6. Divide among 4 bowls, and garnish each bowl with 1 tablespoon Parmesan and ½ tablespoon parsley.

Serving size: 2 ¼ cups pasta

Calories 435; Fat 10g (sat 3g, mono 5g, poly 1g); Cholesterol 17mg; Protein 24g; Carbohydrate 65g; Sugars 8g; Fiber 12g; RS 5g; Sodium 365mg

Resistant Starch 5g

Broccoli & Cheese-Stuffed Baked Potato

PREP: 10 MINUTES
COOK: 13 MINUTES TO 70 MINUTES,
DEPENDING ON METHOD
TOTAL TIME: 23 MINUTES (MICROWAVE)
MAKES: 4 SERVINGS

- 4 Idaho potatoes, scrubbed (10 ounces)
- ¾ cup skim milk
- 1 tablespoon flour
- 4 ounces reduced-fat extra-sharp Cheddar cheese, shredded
- ½ teaspoon salt
- ¼ teaspoon pepper
- ⅛ teaspoon cayenne pepper
- 1 (10-ounce) package frozen broccoli florets, defrosted

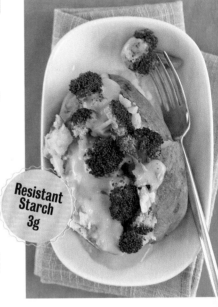

Resistant Starch 3g

1. Cook potatoes:
   OVEN: Preheat oven to 400°. Pierce potatoes with a fork, and wrap each in foil. Bake until tender, 1 hour.
   MICROWAVE: Pierce potatoes with a fork, and wrap each in a paper towel. Place in microwave, and cook on high 8 minutes, until just tender when pierced with a fork (potatoes will continue to cook when removed from microwave).
   While potatoes are cooking, make sauce:
2. Combine milk and flour in a small saucepan, bring to simmer, and cook, whisking, until thickened, 2–3 minutes. Add cheese, salt, pepper, and cayenne, and whisk until sauce is smooth. Continue to simmer, whisking, an additional 2 minutes.
3. Heat broccoli in a heat-safe dish in the microwave for 4–5 minutes, until hot.
4. Split cooked potatoes open with a knife. Spoon ½ cup broccoli into each potato, and top with ¼ cup Cheddar sauce.

Serving size: 1 potato, ½ cup broccoli, and ¼ cup Cheddar sauce | Calories 377; Fat 6g (sat 3g, mono 1g, poly 0g); Cholesterol 17mg; Protein 18g; Carbohydrate 66g; Sugars 6g; Fiber 7g; RS 3g; Sodium 403mg

Pan-Seared Scallops with Southwestern Rice Salad

PREP: 20 MINUTES
COOK: 10 MINUTES
TOTAL TIME: 30 MINUTES
MAKES: 4 SERVINGS

- 1 lime
- 2 teaspoons olive oil, divided
- 1 teaspoon chili powder, divided
- ½ teaspoon salt, divided
- 1 (15-ounce) can low-sodium black beans, rinsed and drained
- 1 (11-ounce) canned corn, drained
- 1 cup grape tomatoes, halved
- ½ cup chopped scallions
- 2 tablespoons chopped fresh cilantro
- 3 cups cooked brown rice
- 1 pound dry scallops (about 16)

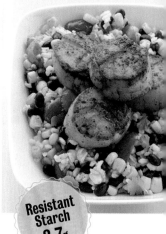

Resistant Starch
3.7g

1. Squeeze juice from half the lime into a large bowl; add 1 teaspoon olive oil, ½ teaspoon chili powder, and ¼ teaspoon salt; stir well with a whisk. Add beans, corn, tomato, scallions, and cilantro; toss gently to combine. Stir in cooked rice, and toss until thoroughly combined. Cover loosely, and keep warm.

2. Combine remaining 1 teaspoon olive oil, remaining ½ teaspoon chili powder, and remaining ¼ teaspoon salt in a large bowl. Pat scallops dry with a paper towel, and add to oil mixture, tossing until thoroughly coated. Squeeze 2 teaspoons juice from remaining lime half into a small bowl, and set aside.

3. Heat a large nonstick skillet over medium-high heat. Arrange scallops in pan, flat sides down (make sure they aren't touching, or they will steam and not sear properly). Cook 2–3 minutes on each side until lightly browned and opaque in the center. Drizzle scallops with reserved lime juice, and toss gently to coat. Divide rice mixture evenly among 4 serving dishes, and top each serving with 4 scallops. Serve immediately.

Serving size: 4 scallops and 1½ cups rice salad | Calories 419; Fat 5g (sat 1g, mono 2g, poly 1g); Cholesterol 37mg; Protein 30g; Carbohydrate 64g; Sugars 4g; Fiber 9g; RS 3.7g; Sodium 497mg

Fish Tacos with Sesame-Ginger Slaw

PREP: 10 MINUTES
COOK: 10 MINUTES
TOTAL TIME: 20 MINUTES
MAKES: 4 SERVINGS

- 1½ pounds tilapia fillets
  Cooking spray
- ¼ teaspoon salt
- ¼ teaspoon pepper
- 3 tablespoons plain, low-fat Greek yogurt
- 2 tablespoons lime juice
- 1 tablespoon dark sesame oil
- 1 tablespoon low-sodium soy sauce
- 2 teaspoons grated, peeled fresh ginger
- 1 teaspoon honey
- 3 cups shredded coleslaw mix
- 12 (6-inch) corn tortillas, warmed

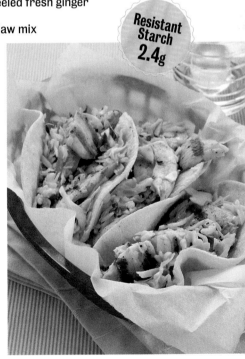

Resistant Starch 2.4g

1. Heat a nonstick skillet or grill pan over medium heat. Coat fish with cooking spray; sprinkle with salt and pepper. Add fish to pan; cook 10–12 minutes, turning once, until fish flakes easily with a fork.
2. Combine yogurt and next 5 ingredients (through honey) in a small bowl, stirring with a whisk. Combine dressing and coleslaw mix, tossing to coat.
3. Flake fish into pieces with a fork. Place 2 ounces fish in each tortilla. Top with coleslaw.

Serving size: 3 tacos | Calories 390; Fat 9g (sat 2g, mono 3g, poly 3g); Cholesterol 85mg; Protein 40g; Carbohydrate 38g; Sugars 4g; Fiber 6g; RS 2.4g; Sodium 430mg

Seared Chicken Breasts with French Potato Salad

PREP: 15 MINUTES
COOK: 20 MINUTES
TOTAL TIME: 35 MINUTES
MAKES: 4 SERVINGS

- 1½ pounds baby Yukon gold potatoes
- 1 cup frozen whole green beans
- 2 tablespoons olive oil, divided
- 2 tablespoons chopped fresh parsley
- 1 tablespoon Dijon mustard
- 1 tablespoon cider vinegar
- ½ teaspoon salt, divided
- Freshly ground black pepper
- 4 (5-ounce) skinless, boneless chicken breasts
- 2 tablespoons all-purpose flour
- 1 large shallot, finely chopped (about ½ cup)
- ¼ cup fresh lemon juice
- 1½ teaspoons dried tarragon

1. Place potatoes in a large saucepan; cover with water. Bring water to a boil, and cook 15 minutes or until potatoes can be easily pierced with a fork. Add green beans during last minute of cooking; drain and set aside.
2. While potatoes and beans cook, combine 1 tablespoon olive oil, parsley, mustard, vinegar, and ¼ teaspoon salt in a large bowl; stir with a whisk. Season to taste with black pepper. When potatoes are cool enough to handle, slice larger pieces in half, and add to bowl. Toss to coat; set aside.
3. Cover chicken breasts with parchment paper; pound to an even thickness using a mallet or heavy skillet. Sprinkle with remaining ¼ teaspoon salt, and season with black pepper.
4. Place flour in a shallow dish; dredge chicken in flour. Heat remaining 1 tablespoon olive oil in a large nonstick skillet over medium-high heat. Add chicken to pan, and cook 6–8 minutes or until chicken begins to brown; turn to brown other side. Add shallots, and cook 5–6 minutes or until a meat thermometer inserted into thickest part of chicken breast registers 165°. Add lemon juice and tarragon, and turn chicken until evenly coated.
5. Place chicken breast on each of 4 serving plates; serve with potato salad.

Serving size: 1 chicken breast and 1¼ cups potato salad | Calories 380; Fat 9g (sat 1.5g, mono 5g, poly 1g); Cholesterol 80mg; Protein 37g; Carbohydrate 37g; Sugars 3g; Fiber 5g; RS 2.3g; Sodium 490mg

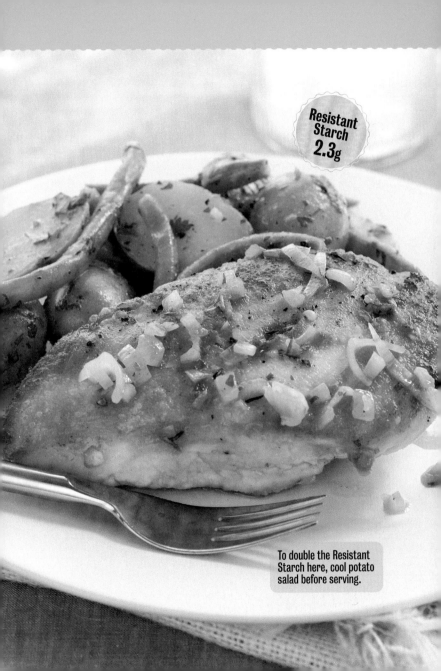

Resistant
Starch
2.3g

To double the Resistant
Starch here, cool potato
salad before serving.

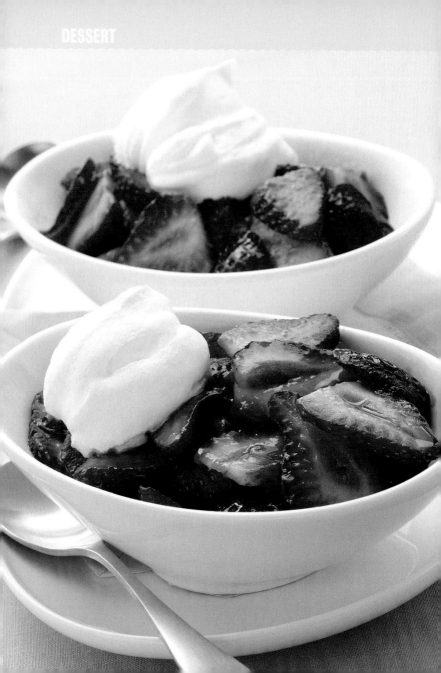

Merlot Strawberries with Whipped Cream

PREP: 5 MINUTES
COOK: 5 MINUTES
TOTAL TIME: 10 MINUTES
MAKES: 4 SERVINGS

- ½ cup merlot
- 2 tablespoons fresh lemon juice
- 2 tablespoons honey
- ¼ teaspoon vanilla extract
- 3 cups sliced strawberries
- 1 cup whipped cream

1. Bring merlot, juice, and honey to a boil in a saucepan over high heat. Remove from heat; stir in vanilla.
2. Drizzle sauce over sliced berries. Top with whipped cream.

Serving size: ¾ cup berries, ¼ cup whipped cream, and 2 tablespoons wine sauce | Calories 140; Fat 3.5g (sat 2g, mono 1g, poly 0.5g); Cholesterol 10mg; Protein 1g; Carbohydrate 22g; Sugars 16g; Fiber 3g; RS 0g; Sodium 20mg

This recipe doesn't have Resistant Starch (RS), but it's packed with fiber and antioxidants. Make sure to get your RS from your other meals, then enjoy this for dessert.

Coconut-Date Truffles

PREP: 10 MINUTES
TOTAL TIME: 10 MINUTES
MAKES: 4 SERVINGS

- 8 dates, pitted and chopped
- 8 tablespoons puffed-wheat cereal
- 2 tablespoons shredded coconut

1. Place dates in a large bowl. Mash with fingers until dates form a ball.
2. Add cereal; knead into dates.
3. Form into 8 balls; roll each in coconut to coat.

Serving size: 2 truffles | Calories 160; Fat 2g (sat 1.5g, mono 0g, poly 0g); Cholesterol 0mg; Protein 1g; Carbohydrate 38g; Sugars 32g; Fiber 4g; RS 0.2g; Sodium 0mg

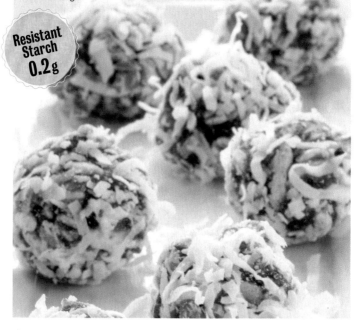

Resistant
Starch
0.2g

Banana Ice Cream

PREP: 5 MINUTES
TOTAL TIME: 5 MINUTES
MAKES: 1 SERVING

 1 small banana, peeled, sliced, and frozen
 3 tablespoons 1% low-fat milk
 1 tablespoon chopped walnuts

1. Place frozen banana pieces and milk in a blender or food processor; process until thick. Top with walnuts.

Serving size: ½ cup | Calories 160; Fat 6g (sat 1g, mono 1g, poly 3.5g); Cholesterol 0mg; Protein 4g; Carbohydrate 26g; Sugars 15g; Fiber 3g; RS 4g; Sodium 20mg

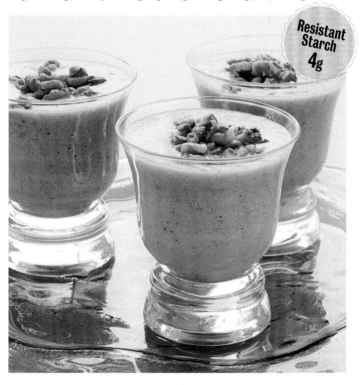

Resistant Starch 4g

Warm Pear with Cinnamon Ricotta

PREP: 5 MINUTES
COOK: 10 MINUTES
TOTAL TIME: 15 MINUTES
MAKES: 1 SERVING

1 small pear, halved and cored
¼ cup part-skim ricotta cheese
¼ teaspoon cinnamon

1. Preheat broiler or toaster oven. Place pear on a baking sheet; broil 10–12 minutes until tender.
2. Combine ricotta and cinnamon in a small bowl. Top warm pear with ricotta mixture.

Serving size: 1 pear and ¼ cup topping | Calories 170; Fat 5g (sat 3g, mono 1.5g, poly 0g); Cholesterol 20mg; Protein 8g; Carbohydrate 27g; Sugars 15g; Fiber 5g; RS 0g; Sodium 80mg

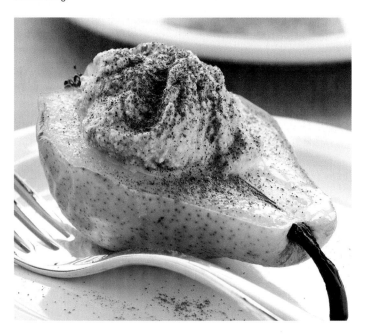

Dark Chocolate & Oat Clusters

PREP: 5 MINUTES
COOK: 3 MINUTES
STAND: 10 MINUTES
TOTAL TIME: 18 MINUTES
MAKES: 4 SERVINGS

- 2 tablespoons peanut butter
- 2 tablespoons 1% low-fat milk
- ¼ cup semisweet chocolate chips
- ¾ cup old-fashioned rolled oats

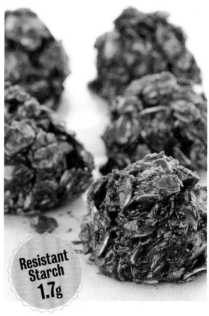

1. Heat peanut butter, milk, and chocolate chips in a saucepan over low heat 3 minutes or until chips melt.
2. Stir in oats. Remove from heat.
3. With a spoon, small ice-cream scoop, or melon baller, drop 8 ball-shaped portions on a baking sheet lined with wax paper. Let set in fridge for 10 minutes before serving.

Resistant Starch 1.7g

Serving size: 2 clusters | Calories 160; Fat 8g (sat 3g, mono 3.5g, poly 1.5g); Cholesterol 0mg; Protein 5g; Carbohydrate 19g; Sugars 7g; Fiber 3g; RS 1.7g; Sodium 40mg

Chocolate-Orange Spoonbread

PREP: 5 MINUTES
COOK: 45 MINUTES
TOTAL TIME: 50 MINUTES
MAKES: 6 SERVINGS

- 1 tablespoon unsalted butter
- ⅓ cup sugar
- ¾ cup fine cornmeal
- 2½ cups cold water
- 3 ounces 70 percent dark chocolate, chopped
- Zest of 1 orange (about 1 teaspoon)
- Orange slices for garnish, optional

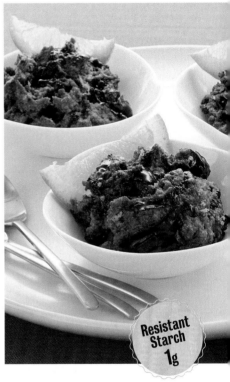

Resistant Starch 1g

1. Preheat oven to 350°.
2. Spread butter along bottom and sides of a 3-quart baking dish. Add sugar, cornmeal, and 2½ cups cold water; stir well with a whisk. Bake at 350° for 30 minutes. Remove from oven, and stir mixture carefully with a fork or whisk until smooth; bake an additional 15 minutes.
3. Remove from oven, and stir until smooth. Add chocolate; stir until chocolate melts completely. Garnish with zest, and serve warm or at room temperature with a slice of orange, if desired.

Serving size: ⅓ cup | Calories 200; Fat 8g (sat 5g, mono 2g, poly 0g); Cholesterol 5mg; Protein 2g; Carbohydrate 29g; Sugars 14g; Fiber 4g; RS 1 g; Sodium 12mg

Chocolate-Dipped Banana Bites

PREP: 5 MINUTES
COOK: 5 MINUTES
TOTAL TIME: 10 MINUTES
MAKES: 1 SERVING

2 tablespoons semisweet chocolate chips
1 small banana, peeled and cut into 1-inch chunks

1. Place chocolate chips in a small microwave-safe bowl. Microwave on HIGH 1 minute or until chocolate melts. Dip banana pieces halfway in melted chocolate. Serve immediately

Serving size: 1 banana | Calories 190; Fat 7g (sat 4g, mono 2g, poly 0.5g); Cholesterol 0mg; Protein 2g; Carbohydrate 36g; Sugars 24g; Fiber 4g; RS 4g; Sodium 0mg

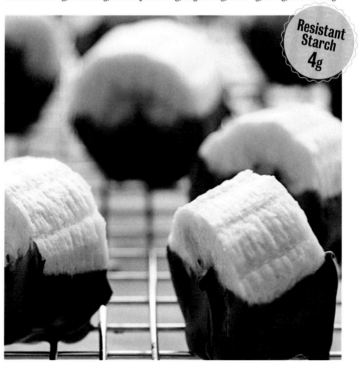

Resistant Starch 4g

Super-Simple CarbLovers Snacks

EASY-TO-MAKE SNACKS ARE KEY TO THE *CARBLOVERS* PLAN. THE 10 snacks listed below can be assembled in minutes and pack about 150 calories each. They keep your energy up between meals and prevent you from overeating all day.

1. Antipasto Platter: On a serving plate, arrange 12 black olives; ½ cup bottled marinated artichoke hearts, drained; and ½ of a bottled roasted red bell pepper, sliced.

2. Pistachio & Dried Cherry Crostini: Combine 2 tablespoons low-fat cottage cheese with 1 teaspoon honey, 2 teaspoons chopped pistachios, and 2 teaspoons chopped dried cherries; serve atop 2 rye crispbread crackers.

3. Brie & Apple Slices: Enjoy 1 small sliced apple with 1 ounce Brie.

4. Cheddar & Apple Melt: Slice 1 small apple and place on a 6-inch corn tortilla. Sprinkle with 1 tablespoon shredded Cheddar cheese. Microwave on HIGH 30 seconds.

5. Greek Yogurt with Orange Marmalade & Walnuts: Combine ½ cup plain low-fat Greek yogurt with 2 teaspoons 100-percent-fruit orange marmalade and 1 tablespoon chopped walnuts.

6. Honey-Curried Yogurt Dip with Carrots & Broccoli: Combine ½ cup plain low-fat Greek yogurt with 1 teaspoon honey, ¼ teaspoon curry powder, and ⅛ teaspoon salt; serve with ½ cup each baby carrots and broccoli florets.

7. Hummus with Feta & Dill: Top 4 tablespoons store-bought hummus with 1 tablespoon feta cheese and ⅛ teaspoon dried dill; serve with 1 cup sliced cucumber.

8. Salmon & Cream Cheese Bites: Spread 2 teaspoons low-fat cream cheese on 1 slice toasted pumpernickel bread; top with ½ ounce smoked salmon and 2 teaspoons chopped chives.

9. Trail Mix: Combine ½ cup cornflakes, 2 tablespoons sliced almonds, and 2 tablespoons dried cherries.

10. White Bean & Herb Hummus with Crudités   Recipe ➡

White Bean & Herb Hummus with Crudités

PREP: 5 MINUTES
TOTAL TIME: 5 MINUTES
MAKES: 1 SERVING

- ¼ cup canned white beans, rinsed and drained
- 1 tablespoon chopped chives
- 1 tablespoon lemon juice
- 2 teaspoons olive oil
- ½ cup assorted raw vegetables, such as chopped broccoli florets, cherry tomatoes, zucchini spears, and sugar snap peas

1. Combine beans, chives, lemon juice, and oil in a small bowl. Mash with a fork until mixture thickens but still has texture.
2. Serve with vegetables.

Serving size: ¼ cup hummus and ½ cup raw vegetables | Calories 150; Fat 10g (sat 1.5g, mono 7g, poly 1g); Cholesterol 0mg; Protein 4g; Carbohydrate 14g; Sugars 3g; Fiber 3g; RS 2g; Sodium 35mg

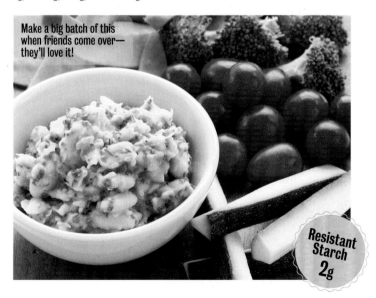

Make a big batch of this when friends come over— they'll love it!

Resistant Starch 2g

Supermarket Choices

For the healthiest, tastiest ingredients, packaged meals, and treats, look for these *CarbLovers*-approved brands!

Nutritional information is per individual portion. Check labels for portion size.	CALORIES	FAT	FIBER	CARBS	SODIUM
BREAD					
Arnold Sandwich Thins Seedless Rye	100	1	5	23	210
Arnold Natural Flax & Fiber	100	2	5	21	170
Aunt Millie's Healthy Goodness Fiber & Flavor Potato Bread	120	1.5	3	24	250
Aunt Millie's Healthy Goodness Whole Grain White Bread	95	1.5	5	21	180
Aunt Millie's Fiber for Life Light Five Grain Bread	80	1	5	20	180
Aunt Millie's Hearth Whole Grain Hamburger Buns	140	2	3	27	310
Ener-G Foods Corn Loaf	40	2	3	7	50
Ener-G Foods Seattle Hamburger & Hot Dog Buns	160	4.5	8	35	190
Ener-G Foods Brown English Muffins with Flax	180	5	7	35	250
Flatout Original Light wraps	90	2.5	9	16	320
Food for Life Ezekiel 4:9 Organic Sprouted 100% Whole Grain Flourless Bread	80	0.5	3	15	75
Food for Life Genesis 1:29 Organic Sprouted Grain & Seed Bread	80	2	3	14	65
Food for Life Organic 7-Sprouted 100% Whole Grain Flourless Bread	80	0.5	3	15	80
Food for Life Organic 7-Sprouted 100% Whole Grain Flourless English Muffins	80	1	3	16	120
Food for Life Ezekiel 4:9 Organic 100% Whole Grain Pita Pocket Bread	100	0.1	4	21	120
Food for Life Whole Grain Spelt Bread	110	2	3	20	160

	CALORIES	FAT	FIBER	CARBS	SODIUM
Food for Life Ezekiel 4:9 Organic Sprouted 100% Whole Grain Flourless Sesame Burger Buns	170	1.5	6	32	180
French Meadow Sprouted Cinnamon Raisin Bread	100	0.5	3	19	80
French Meadow Sprouted 16 Grain & Seed Bread	110	2.5	4	17	80
French Meadow Sprouted Grain Bread	100	0.5	4	18	85
French Meadow Sprouted 16 Grain & Seed Bagel	250	2.5	10	42	220
French Meadow Sprouted Cinnamon Raisin Bagel	270	1.5	7	50	270
French Meadow Sprouted Grain Tortilla	150	0.5	5	27	160
La Tortilla Factory Whole Wheat 100-Calorie Tortilla Wraps	100	1.5	8	24	320
La Tortilla Factory Extra Virgin Olive Oil Tomato Basil SoftWraps	100	3	12	20	360
Storye Classic Rye Bread	145	1	8	44	221
Storye Fine Rye Bread	157	1	6	47	201
Storye Classic Rye Bread with Carrots	155	1	6	46	274
Storye Fine Rye Bread with Fruit and Nuts	170	5	6	43	158
BREAKFAST					
Boca Breakfast Links	70	3	2	5	330
Kellogg's Eggo Real Fruit Pizza Mixed Berry Granola	390	13	4	62	390
Kellogg's Eggo Real Fruit Pizza Strawberry Granola	400	12	4	66	390
Thomas' 100% Whole Wheat Bagel Thins	110	1	5	24	190
Thomas' 100% Whole Wheat English Muffins	120	1	3	23	220
Thomas' Light Multi-Grain English Muffins	100	1	8	26	180
CAKE					
Wellness Bakeries Chocolate Bliss Cake Mix	178	3	7	21	126
CEREAL					
Barbara's Bakery High Fiber Original	180	1.5	14	42	140

	CALORIES	FAT	FIBER	CARBS	SODIUM
Barbara's Bakery High Fiber Flax & Granola	200	3	10	42	140
Barbara's Bakery High Fiber Cranberry	190	1.5	10	42	140
Barbara's Bakery Shredded Spoonfuls Multigrain	120	1.5	4	24	200
Barbara's Bakery Cinnamon Puffins	90	1	6	26	150
Barbara's Bakery Honey Rice Puffins	120	1	3	25	80
Barbara's Bakery Multigrain Puffins	110	0	3	25	80
Bear Naked 100% Pure & Natural Granola Peak Protein	140	7	3	15	25
Bear Naked 100% Pure & Natural Cereal Banana Nut	220	5	7	43	210
Bob's Red Mill Organic High Fiber Cereal	150	5	10	27	0
Bob's Red Mill Gluten-Free Quick Rolled Oats	180	3	5	29	0
Cascadian Farm Hearty Morning Cereal	200	3	8	43	360
Cheerios Oat Cluster Crunch	100	1	4	22	135
Fiber One Original Cereal	60	1	14	25	105
Food for Life Ezekiel 4:9 Organic Sprouted 100% Whole Grain Flourless Almond Cereal	200	3	6	38	190
Food for Life Ezekiel 4:9 Organic Sprouted 100% Whole Grain Flourless Golden Flax Cereal	180	2.5	6	37	190
GrandyOats Granola Mainely Maple	204	7	4	31	109
Kashi Good Friends Cereal	160	1.5	12	42	110
Kashi GoLean Cereal	140	1	10	30	85
Kashi GoLean Crisp Toasted Blueberry Crumble	180	3.5	8	35	125
Kashi GoLean Crunch Honey Almond Flax	200	4.5	8	36	140
Kellogg's All-Bran Original Cereal	80	1	10	23	80
Kellogg's Corn Flakes	100	0	1	24	200
Mona's Original Granola	140	7	3	16	0
Nature's Path Optimum Banana Almond	190	6	5	35	140
Nature's Path Optimum Cranberry Ginger	190	2.5	8	41	95
Nature's Path Flax Plus Flakes	110	1.5	5	23	135
Nature's Path Heritage Flakes	120	1	5	24	130
Nature's Path Mesa Sunrise Flakes	120	1	3	24	125

	CALORIES	FAT	FIBER	CARBS	SODIUM
Nature's Path Crunchy Maple Sunrise	110	1	3	25	130
Nature's Path Crunchy Vanilla Sunrise	110	1	3	25	130
Nature's Path Millet Rice Flakes	120	2	3	22	115
Nature's Path Multigrain Oatbran Flakes	110	1	5	24	110
Nature's Path SmartBran	90	1	13	24	130
Nature's Path Whole O's	110	1.5	3	25	115
Nature's Path Pumpkin Flax Plus Granola	260	10	5	37	45
Nature's Path Hemp Plus Granola	260	10	5	36	45
Nature's Path Peanut Butter Granola	260	11	4	35	75
Nature's Path Pomegran Plus Granola	250	9	4	38	60
Nature's Path Vanilla Almond Flax Plus Granola	250	9	5	36	80
Nature's Path Agave Plus Granola	250	9	4	37	95
Post Grape Nuts	200	1	7	48	290
Post Shredded Wheat	160	1	6	37	0
Post Raisin Bran	190	1	8	46	250
Post Trail Mix Crunch	180	2.5	5	37	210
CHIPS					
Beanitos Black Bean chips	140	7	5	15	55
Beanitos Pinto Bean & Flax chips	140	8	5	15	55
Beanitos Pinto Bean & Flax with Cheddar Cheese chips	140	8	5	14	140
Beanitos Black Bean with BBQ chips	140	7	5	15	150
Corazonas Lightly Salted Tortilla Chips	140	7	3	18	75
Corazonas Squeeze of Lime Tortilla Chips	140	7	3	17	140
Corazonas Parmesan Peppercorn Potato Chips	140	6	2	18	160
Corazonas Spicy Rio Habanero Potato Chips	130	6	2	18	120
Flatout Garlic Herb crisps	120	4	5	16	330
Flatout Four Cheese crisps	130	4.5	5	15	290
Flatout Multigrain crisps	120	4	5	16	240
Food Should Taste Good Multigrain chips	140	6	3	18	80
Newman's Own Organics Soy Crisps Barbeque	110	3.5	3	14	390

	CALORIES	FAT	FIBER	CARBS	SODIUM
Newman's Own Organics Soy Crisps Cinnamon Sugar	120	4	3	15	170
Newman's Own Organics Soy Crisps White Cheddar	120	4	3	13	290
COUSCOUS					
Near East Whole Grain Blends Wheat Couscous: Roasted Garlic & Olive Oil	190	2.5	3	37	510
CRACKERS					
Archer Farms Simply Balanced Snack Crackers: Sun-Dried Tomato & Basil	130	3	2	24	220
Back to Nature Whole Wheat Crackers	120	4.5	3	19	140
Kashi TLC Party Crackers Mediterranean Bruschetta	120	4	3	18	140
Kashi TLC Party Crackers Roasted Garlic & Thyme	130	4.5	3	18	140
Kashi TLC Party Crackers Stoneground 7 Grain	130	5	3	17	130
Triscuit Original Crackers	120	4.5	3	19	180
Triscuit Hint of Salt Crackers	130	5	3	19	50
Triscuit Rosemary & Olive Oil Crackers	120	4	3	20	135
Wasa Thin & Crispy Flatbread Original	70	1.5	1	12	130
Wasa Thin & Crispy Flatbread Sesame	70	2	1	11	100
Wasa Thin & Crispy Flatbread Rosemary	70	1.5	1	12	180
Wasa Fiber Crispbread Crackers	35	0.5	2	8	60
Wheat Thins Fiber Selects	120	4.5	5	22	260
DRIED FRUIT					
Mariani Enhanced Wellness Berry Thrive with Omega-3 Dried Fruit	140	0	2	32	0
EGGS					
Eggland's Best Organic Eggs	70	4	0	0	60
FROZEN FOOD (BREAKFAST)					
Amy's Kitchen Breakfast Burrito	270	8	5	38	540
Amy's Kitchen Breakfast Scramble Wrap	380	19	4	30	490
Amy's Kitchen Multi-Grain Hot Cereal Bowl	190	1.5	5	40	300
Amy's Kitchen Steel-Cut Oats Hot Cereal Bowl	220	3.5	5	42	190

	CALORIES	FAT	FIBER	CARBS	SODIUM
Amy's Kitchen Tofu Scramble	320	19	4	19	580
Bob Evans Cranberry Pecan Oatmeal Bowl	290	7	5	53	490
Bob Evans Hearty Blueberry Oatmeal Bowl	240	3.5	5	50	490
Jimmy Dean D-Lights Turkey Bacon Breakfast Bowl	240	9	2	20	760
Lean Pockets Applewood Bacon, Egg & Cheese	290	8	2	40	480
Smart Ones Breakfast Quesadilla	230	7	6	29	730
Smart Ones Stuffed Breakfast Sandwich	240	7	3	30	570

	CALORIES	FAT	FIBER	CARBS	SODIUM
Amy's Kitchen Brown Rice, Black-Eyed Peas & Veggies Bowl	290	11	8	38	580
Amy's Kitchen Baked Ziti Bowl	390	12	6	62	590
Amy's Kitchen Brown Rice & Vegetables Bowl, light in sodium	260	9	5	36	270
Amy's Kitchen Mexican Casserole Bowl, light in sodium	370	16	7	48	390
Amy's Kitchen Baked Ziti Kids Meal	350	12	4	57	460
Amy's Kitchen Indian Paneer Tikka	320	19	5	36	550
Amy's Kitchen Indian Mattar Paneer, light in sodium	320	8	6	54	390
Amy's Kitchen Asian Noodle Stir-Fry	300	7	5	50	630
Amy's Kitchen Thai Stir-Fry	310	11	5	45	420
Amy's Kitchen Veggie Loaf Whole Meal, light in sodium	290	8	10	47	340
Amy's Kitchen Light & Lean Spinach Lasagna	260	4	5	40	540
Amy's Kitchen Light & Lean Pasta & Veggies	210	5	3	33	470
Amy's Kitchen Light & Lean Soft Shell Taco Fiesta	210	4.5	5	40	560
Amy's Kitchen Light & Lean Black Bean & Cheese Enchilada	240	4.5	4	44	480
Amy's Kitchen Indian Spinach Tofu Wrap	270	13	6	28	690
Amy's Kitchen Southwestern Burrito	290	10	6	38	680
Amy's Kitchen Chili & Cornbread Whole Meal	340	6	10	59	680

	CALORIES	FAT	FIBER	CARBS	SODIUM
Amy's Kitchen Black Bean Enchilada Whole Meal with Spanish Rice and Beans	330	8	9	53	740
Amy's Kitchen Black Bean Vegetable Enchiladas	160	6	3	22	390
Dr. Praeger's Pizza Bagel	110	2.5	3	16	180
Dr. Praeger's Falafel Flats	110	4.5	4	14	135
Dr. Praeger's Burrito Bites	130	3	4	20	210
Dr. Praeger's California Veggie Balls	80	2.5	3	10	190
Dr. Praeger's California Veggie Pockets	150	5	5	22	240
Ethnic Gourmet Pad Thai with Tofu	420	8	3	73	720
Ethnic Gourmet Lemongrass & Basil Chicken	380	9	5	56	310
Ethnic Gourmet Malay Chicken Curry	410	11	3	59	530
Ethnic Gourmet Chicken Korma	340	9	3	44	720
Evol Cilantro Lime Chicken Burrito	320	7	4	49	450
Evol Veggie Fajita Burrito	290	3.5	5	56	440
Evol Basic Bean & Cheese Burrito	360	7	8	60	620
Evol Tofu & Spinach Sauté Burrito	300	5	6	52	510
Guiltless Gourmet California Veggie Wrap	230	7	6	40	470
Guiltless Gourmet Mediterranean Spinach Wrap	220	6	6	39	410
Guiltless Gourmet Black Bean Chipotle Wrap	230	6	7	47	450
Healthy Choice Oven Roasted Chicken	250	5	5	35	540
Healthy Choice Café Steamers Chicken Pesto Classico	310	8	4	38	530
Healthy Choice Café Steamers Chicken Margherita	330	8	4	42	500
Healthy Choice Café Steamers Grilled Basil Chicken	270	6	7	34	600
Healthy Choice Café Steamers Lemon Garlic Chicken and Shrimp	260	6	6	35	600
Healthy Choice Café Steamers Grilled Vegetables Mediterranean	220	2.5	7	42	600
Healthy Choice Honey Balsamic Chicken	220	3.5	5	34	540

	CALORIES	FAT	FIBER	CARBS	SODIUM
Kashi Black Bean Mango	340	8	7	58	340
Kashi Chicken Pasta Pomodoro	280	6	6	38	470
Kashi Chicken Florentine	290	9	5	31	550
Kashi Lemongrass Coconut Chicken	300	8	7	38	680
Kashi Mayan Harvest Bake	340	9	8	58	380
Kashi Pesto Pasta Primavera	290	11	7	37	750
Kashi Red Curry Chicken	300	8	6	42	420
Kashi Southwest Style Chicken	310	5	6	49	680
Kashi Sweet and Sour Chicken	320	3.5	6	55	380
Kashi Tuscan Veggie Bake	260	9	8	42	700
Kashi Veggie Chana Masala	310	9	8	44	690
Lean Cuisine Sun Dried Tomato Pesto Chicken	270	9	4	28	570
Lean Cuisine Ginger Garlic Stir Fry with Chicken	280	4	5	42	550
Lean Cuisine Salmon with Basil	220	6	5	26	600
Lean Pockets Whole Grain Turkey, Broccoli & Cheese	260	8	4	38	430
Lean Pockets Whole Grain Culinary Creations Grilled Chicken, Mushroom & Spinach	240	6	3	38	480
Lean Pockets Whole Grain Culinary Creations Chipotle Chicken	260	7	4	39	530
Palermo's Primo Thin Garden Pizza	270	12	3	28	780
Palermo's Primo Thin Fajita Pizza	250	12	2	21	530
Palermo's Primo Thin Margherita Pizza	260	12	2	26	660
FROZEN SIDES					
Amy's Kitchen Organic Vegetarian Baked Beans	140	0.5	6	28	480
Amy's Kitchen Organic Traditional Refried Beans	140	3	6	22	390
Alexia Sweet Potato Julienne Fries	140	5	3	24	140
Alexia Spicy Sweet Potato Julienne Fries	130	4	3	23	250
Birds Eye Steamfresh Broccoli, Cauliflower & Carrots	30	0	2	5	30

	CALORIES	FAT	FIBER	CARBS	SODIUM
Dr. Praeger's Potato Pancakes	100	4	3	13	190
Dr. Praeger's Sweet Potato Pancakes	80	2	3	12	140
FROZEN TREATS					
Häagen-Dazs Chocolate Lowfat Sorbet	130	0.5	2	28	70
Skinny Cow Fudge Bars	100	1	4	22	45
Skinny Cow Chocolate Peanut Butter Low Fat Sandwich	150	2	3	30	100
HOT CEREAL					
Bob's Red Mill 7 Grain Hot Cereal	140	1.5	6	28	0
Country Choice Organic Old Fashioned Oats	150	3	4	27	0
Country Choice Organic Quick Oats	150	3	4	27	0
Country Choice Organic Multigrain Hot Cereal	130	1	5	29	0
Country Choice Organic Steel Cut Oats	150	3	4	27	0
Country Choice Organic Maple Instant Oatmeal	170	2	3	32	60
Country Choice Organic Apple Cinnamon Instant Oatmeal	140	1.5	3	22	60
Country Choice Organic Original Instant Oatmeal	110	2	3	19	0
Hodgson Mill Multi Grain Hot Cereal with Flaxseed and Soy	160	3	6	25	0
Nature's Path Apple Cinnamon Hot Oatmeal	210	2.5	4	40	100
Nature's Path Flax Plus Hot Oatmeal	210	3	5	38	140
Nature's Path Hemp Plus Hot Oatmeal	160	2.5	4	30	105
Nature's Path Maple Nut Hot Oatmeal	210	4	4	38	100
Nature's Path MultiGrain Raisin Spice Oatmeal	180	1	4	39	100
Nature's Path Optimum Cinnamon, Blueberry, and Flaxseed Oatmeal	150	2.5	3	29	115
Quaker Hearty Medleys Apple Cranberry Almond	130	2.5	3	27	135
JUICE					
Tropicana Healthy Heart Orange Juice with Omega-3	120	0.5	0	26	0

	CALORIES	FAT	FIBER	CARBS	SODIUM
MILK					
Smart Balance Fat-Free Milk with Omega-3s and Vitamin E	110	1	0	14	150
MUFFINS					
Aunt Millie's Whole Grain Blueberry Muffins	170	8	3	23	150
Aunt Millie's Whole Grain Brownie Muffins	220	9	2	35	130
Aunt Millie's Whole Grain Chocolate Chip Muffins	190	9	3	23	150
Aunt Millie's Whole Grain Coffee Cake Muffins	190	9	3	26	150
Fiber One Blueberry Muffins	180	4	7	33	190
Vitalicious VitaMuffins Deep Chocolate	100	1.5	9	26	140
Vitalicious VitaMuffins CranBran	100	0	5	22	140
Vitalicious VitaMuffins Golden Corn	100	1	6	25	135
Vitalicious VitaMuffins BlueBran	100	0	5	20	140
Vitalicious VitaTops Banana Nut	100	2	8	22	105
Vitalicious VitaTops Apple Crumb	100	1	8	25	105
Vitalicious VitaTops Fudgy Peanut Butter Chip	100	1.5	8	26	105
OTHER					
Hellman's Mayonnaise with Extra Virgin Olive Oil	50	5	0	<1	120
King Arthur Flour Hi-Maize Natural Fiber	15	0	6	9	0
King Arthur Flour Hi-Maize High Fiber Flour	90	0	5	23	0
Kraft Mayo with Olive Oil	45	4	0	2	95
Land O' Lakes Butter with Olive Oil	90	10	0	0	90
Olivio Premium Spread Original	80	8	0	0	100
PACKAGED MEAL					
Annie Chun's Pad Thai Brown Rice Noodles	200	1	4	44	10
Annie Chun's Maifun Brown Rice Noodles	200	1	4	44	10
Archer Farms Simply Balanced Lemon & Pepper Fusilli	240	2	4	48	470
Archer Farms Simply Balanced Red Pepper Penne	250	2	7	49	460

	CALORIES	FAT	FIBER	CARBS	SODIUM
Archer Farms Simply Balanced Dinner Kit: Tex Mex Beans & Cornbread Entree	300	2	13	60	570
Archer Farms Simply Balanced Dinner Kit: Garlic Ranch Primavera Entree	190	1	4	39	560
Archer Farms Simply Balanced Garlic & Ranch Primavera Entree	190	1	4	39	560
Archer Farms Simply Balanced Cajun Rice & Beans Entree	210	1.5	8	43	430
Archer Farms Simply Balanced Cajun Style Beans & Rice Lunch Bowl	250	1	9	51	430
Bumble Bee Sensations Seasoned Lemon & Pepper Tuna Medley Kit	110	3	0	2	350
StarKist Charlie's Lunch Kit Chunk Light	210	8	2	19	580
PASTA					
Annie's Lower Sodium Mac and Cheese	270	4	2	47	430
Annie's Organic 5 Grain Elbows & White Cheddar	260	4	3	46	570
Annie's Bunny Pasta with Yummy Cheese	260	3.5	3	46	400
Annie's Penne Pasta with Alfredo	220	3.5	2	37	430
Annie's Curly Fettuccine with White Cheddar & Broccoli Sauce	200	2.5	2	37	450
Archer Farms Simply Balanced Whole Wheat Pasta	200	1	4	43	0
Barilla Plus Pasta	210	2	4	38	25
Barilla Whole Grain	200	1.5	6	41	0
Dreamfields Pasta (spaghetti)	190	1	5	41	10
Racconto Essentials 8 Grain Whole Grain Pasta	190	1	7	42	0
Racconto Essentials Glycemic Health Whole Grain Pasta	190	1	11	42	10
Ronzoni Healthy Harvest Whole Wheat Penne Rigate	180	1	6	41	0
Ronzoni Healthy Harvest Whole Wheat Lasagna	180	1.5	7	39	0
Ronzoni Healthy Harvest Whole Wheat Linguine	180	1	6	41	0

	CALORIES	FAT	FIBER	CARBS	SODIUM
Ronzoni Healthy Harvest Whole Wheat Rotini	180	1	6	41	0
Ronzoni Healthy Harvest Whole Wheat Spaghetti	180	1	6	41	0
Ronzoni Smart Taste	180	0.5	7	43	5
RICE					
Near East Whole Grain Blends Brown Rice Pilaf	180	1	3	41	600
Near East Whole Grain Blends Roasted Garlic	190	2	5	41	510
Near East Whole Grain Blends Roasted Pecan and Garlic	220	5	4	38	480
Near East Creative Grains Mix Creamy Parmesan	240	3	3	49	690
Uncle Ben's Whole Grain Boil-in-Bag Brown Rice	170	1.5	2	36	0
SNACKS					
Annie's Whole Wheat Cheddar Bunnies	130	6	3	17	250
Annie's Chocolate Bunny Grahams; Honey Bunny Grahams	130	4.5	2	21	75
Archer Farms Simply Balanced Peach Mango Fruit & Yogurt Bars	90	0.5	2	21	10
Archer Farms Simply Balanced Strawberry Banana Fruit & Yogurt Bars	110	0.5	3	29	0
Archer Farms Simply Balanced Granola Bars: Blueberry Almond Flax	150	3	4	26	40
Baked Lay's potato chips	120	2	2	23	180
Clif Chocolate Chip Crunch Bar	180	8	3	27	105
Clif Honey Oat Crunch Bar	180	7	3	27	110
Clif Peanut Butter Crunch Bar	190	9	3	25	115
Clif White Chocolate Macadamia Nut Crunch Bar	190	9	3	26	105
Clif Kid ZBar Blueberry	120	2.5	3	23	90
Ener-G Foods Wylde Pretzels	130	3	3	24	230
Evol Mini Burritos Bean & Cheddar	190	3.5	4	32	360

	CALORIES	FAT	FIBER	CARBS	SODIUM
Evol Mini Burritos Veggie Fajita	160	2	3	30	280
Extend Snacks ExtendBar Sugar-Free Chocolate Delight	150	3	6	20	200
Fiber One Oats and Caramel	140	3.5	9	30	105
Fiber One Oats and Strawberry with Almonds	140	3	9	29	90
Fiber One Oats and Peanut Butter	150	4.5	9	28	105
Fiber One Oats and Chocolate	140	4	9	29	95
Hershey's Kisses Special Dark Mildly Sweet Chocolates	180	12	3	25	15
Kashi TLC Cereal Bars Baked Apple Spice	110	3	3	21	105
Kashi TLC Cereal Bars Blackberry Graham	110	3	3	21	125
Kashi TLC Cereal Bars Ripe Strawberry	110	3	3	21	105
Kashi TLC Chewy Granola Bars Cherry Dark Chocolate	120	2	4	24	65
Kashi TLC Chewy Granola Bars Honey Almond Flax	140	5	4	19	105
Kashi TLC Chewy Granola Bars Peanut Peanut Butter	140	5	4	19	85
Kashi TLC Chewy Granola Bars Trail Mix	140	5	4	20	95
Kashi TLC Fruit & Grain Bars Cranberry Walnut	120	3	4	22	50
Kashi TLC Crunchy Granola Bars Pumpkin Spice Flax	170	6	4	26	140
Kashi TLC Crunchy Granola Bars Honey Toasted 7 Grain	170	5	4	26	150
Kashi GoLean Crunch Chocolate Almond Protein & Fiber Bar	170	5	5	27	210
Kashi GoLean Crunch Chocolate Pretzel Protein & Fiber Bar	160	3	5	28	250
Kashi GoLean Crunch Chocolate Caramel Protein & Fiber Bar	150	3	6	28	220
Kashi TLC Cookies Oatmeal Raisin Flax	130	4.5	4	20	70
Kashi TLC Cookies Happy Trail Mix	140	5	4	21	75
Kashi TLC Cookies Oatmeal Dark Chocolate	130	5	4	20	65

	CALORIES	FAT	FIBER	CARBS	SODIUM
Kellogg's FiberPlus Antioxidants Dark Chocolate Almond Bar	130	5	9	24	50
Kellogg's FiberPlus Antioxidants Chocolate Chip Bar	120	4	9	26	55
Kellogg's FiberPlus Antioxidants Chocolatey Peanut Butter Bar	130	5	9	24	95
Kind Cranberry Almond + Antioxidants snack bar	190	13	3	20	20
Kind Peanut Butter Dark Chocolate + Protein snack bar	180	12	2	17	65
Kind Blueberry Pecan + Fiber snack bar	180	10	5	23	25
Lärabar Cherry Pie mini bar	90	4	2	14	0
Laughing Cow Mini Babybel Cheddar cheese	70	5	0	0	140
Laughing Cow Mini Babybel Original cheese	70	6	0	0	170
Laughing Cow Mini Babybel Bonbel cheese	70	6	0	0	170
Laughing Cow Mini Babybel Gouda cheese	80	6	0	0	170
Laughing Cow Mini Babybel Light cheese	50	3	0	0	160
Laughing Cow Light Creamy Swiss wedges	35	1.5	0	1	210
Laughing Cow Light Garlic & Herb wedges	35	1.5	0	1	210
Laughing Cow Light French Onion wedges	35	1.5	0	1	210
Laughing Cow Light Blue Cheese wedges	35	1.5	0	2	230
Laughing Cow Light Mozzarella, Sun-Dried Tomato & Basil wedges	35	2	0	2	220
Laughing Cow Light Queso Fresco & Chipotle wedges	35	1.5	0	2	240
Luna Protein Chocolate Peanut Butter Bar	190	9	3	19	210
Luna Protein Cookie Dough Bar	180	6	3	21	230
Luna Protein Chocolate Cherry Bar Almond	180	7	3	21	105
Nature's Path Sunny Hemp Granola Bar	140	3.5	3	24	90
Nature Valley Sweet & Salty Nut Almond Granola Bar	160	7	2	22	150
Nature Valley Fruit & Nut Trail Mix Bar	140	4	1	25	100

	CALORIES	FAT	FIBER	CARBS	SODIUM
Nature Valley Peanut Butter Crunchy Granola Bar	190	7	2	28	180
Nature Valley Oats 'n Honey Crunchy Granola Bar	190	6	2	29	160
Newman's Own Organics Spelt Pretzels	120	1	4	23	240
Newman's Own Organics Hi-Protein Pretzels	120	1.5	4	22	230
Newman's Own Organics Honey Wheat Pretzels	110	1	3	22	180
Newman's Own Organics Thin Stick Pretzels	110	1.5	4	22	180
Newman's Own Organics Dried Apricots	110	0	2	25	0
Newman's Own Organics Dried Apple Rings	120	0	2	29	0
Nutri-Grain Blueberry, Strawberry, or Blackberry Bar	120	3	3	24	135
Odwalla Banana Nut Bar	220	5	5	39	105
Odwalla Blueberry Swirl Bar	200	3	4	41	125
Quaker Fiber & Omega-3 Peanut Butter Chocolate Granola Bars	150	5	9	25	35
Quaker Oatmeal-to-Go High Fiber Maple Brown Sugar	210	4	10	43	230
Sabra Classic Single Serving Hummus	140	12	2	8	240
Sahale Snacks Soledad Almonds	130	9	3	10	60
Sahale Snacks Barbeque Almonds with Mild Chipotle and Ranch	140	11	3	8	270
Sahale Snacks Tuscan Almonds with Parmesan and Herbs	140	11	3	8	250
Seapoint Farms KooLoos: Original	140	5	3	15	280
Seapoint Farms Dry Roasted Edamame: Lightly Salted	130	4	8	10	150
Soyjoy Banana bar	130	6	2	16	45
Sun-Maid Mediterranean Apricots	100	0	3	23	15
Sun-Maid California Apricots	100	0	3	26	0
Sun-Maid Pitted Plums	100	0	3	26	0
Sun-Maid Mixed Fruit	100	0	3	26	35
Sun-Maid California Mission Figs	120	0	5	28	0

	CALORIES	FAT	FIBER	CARBS	SODIUM
SOUP					
Amy's Kitchen Organic Lentil	180	5	6	25	590
Amy's Kitchen Organic Lentil Vegetable, light in sodium	160	4	8	24	340
Amy's Kitchen Organic Lentil, light in sodium	180	5	6	25	290
Amy's Kitchen Organic Split Pea, light in sodium	100	0	6	19	330
Amy's Kitchen Organic Medium Chili with Vegetables	230	6	9	34	590
Amy's Kitchen Organic Medium Chili, light in sodium	280	9	6	28	480
Amy's Kitchen Organic Spicy Chili, light in sodium	280	9	7	35	340
Campbell's Chunky Healthy Request Vegetable	120	1	4	24	410
Campbell's Select Harvest Chicken Tuscany	90	1.5	4	12	480
Campbell's Select Harvest Light Roasted Chicken with Italian Herbs	80	2.5	3	9	480
Pacific Foods Organic Light Sodium Butternut Squash	90	2	3	17	280
Progresso High Fiber Homestyle Minestrone	110	2	7	24	690
Progresso High Fiber Creamy Tomato Basil	130	4	7	26	690
Progresso High Fiber Hearty Vegetable and Noodle	90	1.5	7	18	690
Progresso High Fiber Three Bean Chili with Beef	140	4	7	23	480
Progresso High Fiber Chicken Tuscany	130	3	7	20	690
VEGGIE BURGER					
Boca Veggie Patties: Bruschetta Tomato Basil Parmesan	90	1.5	5	9	440
Boca Original Vegan Meatless Burger	70	0.5	4	6	280

	CALORIES	FAT	FIBER	CARBS	SODIUM
Dr. Praeger's Bombay Veggie Burgers	110	5	4	13	250
Dr. Praeger's California Veggie Burgers	110	5	4	13	250
Dr. Praeger's Italian Veggie Burgers	110	5	5	13	250
Dr. Praeger's Tex Mex Veggie Burgers	110	4.5	5	13	250
WAFFLES					
Kellogg's Eggo Nutri-Grain Whole Wheat Waffles	170	6	3	26	400
Kellogg's Eggo Nutri-Grain Blueberry Waffles	180	5	3	31	370
YOGURT					
Chobani Non-Fat Plain Greek Yogurt (6 oz)	100	0	0	7	80
Dannon Activia Peach & Cereal Fiber Yogurt (4 oz)	110	2	3	20	60
Fage Total 0% Plain Greek Yogurt (6 oz)	90	0	0	7	65
Stonyfield Oikos Organic Plain Greek Yogurt (5.3 oz)	80	0	0	6	60
Yoplait Fiber One Yogurt (all flavors) (4 oz)	50	0	5	13	55

Restaurant Choices

What's the best dish to order at your favorite dining out spot?
These top *CarbLovers* picks will fill you up—without filling you out!

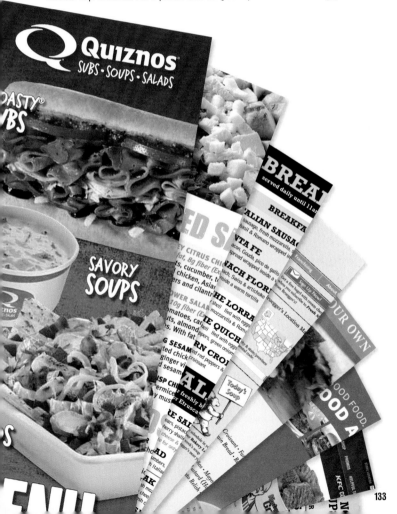

	CALORIES	FAT	FIBER	CARBS	SODIUM
APPLEBEE'S					
Applebee's House Salad (without dressing)	230	15	2	12	390
ARBY'S					
Chicken Sandwich-Roast	400	16	3	40	870
AU BON PAIN					
Apple Cinnamon Oatmeal (medium)	280	4	7	56	10
Oatmeal (medium)	260	5	6	47	10
Apples, Blue Cheese, and Cranberries	200	10	3	27	270
Hummus and Cucumber	130	8	3	10	460
Mayan Chicken Harvest Rice Bowl with Brown Rice (¾ of bowl)	383	9.8	3	54	653
BAJA FRESH					
Original Baja Taco Chicken	210	5	2	28	230
Original Baja Taco Shrimp	200	5	2	28	280
Original Baja Taco Carnitas	220	7	2	29	280
Americano Soft Taco Mahi Mahi	240	10	2	20	490
Americano Soft Taco Steak	260	13	2	21	640
BRUEGGER'S					
Garden Veggie Sandwich on Wheat Bread	360	3	4	67	540
Garden Veggie Sandwich on Plain Bagel	360	2	5	72	550
Spinach and Lentil Soup (8 oz)	110	3.5	7	16	570
White Chicken Chili (8 oz)	240	9	7	26	630
BURGER KING					
Garden Salad (no chicken)	140	6	3	16	220
CHILI'S					
Loaded Baked Potato Soup (cup)	210	15	1	11	590
Terlingua Chili with Toppings (cup)	180	10	3	9	590
CHIPOTLE					
Crispy Tacos with Fajita Vegetables and Guacamole	350	19.5	10	39	390
Burrito Bowl with Chicken, Fajita Vegetables, and Black Beans	330	8	12	28	790

	CALORIES	FAT	FIBER	CARBS	SODIUM
CORNER BAKERY					
Chilled Swiss Oatmeal	360	3	5	78	130
Fresh Berry Parfait	380	12	7	64	160
COSÌ					
Oatmeal	222	3	4	45	98
Fire-Roasted Veggie Sandwich	324	8	4	44	259
Tuscan Pesto Chicken Sandwich	510	6	4	49	452
Signature Salad Light	371	19	5	45	485
Hummus & Fresh Veggies Sandwich	397	7	7	72	532
DENNY'S					
Seasonal Fruit	70	0	3	18	7
Grits with Margarine	220	3	3	44	15
Oatmeal with 8-oz milk	290	8	4	39	300
Veggie-Cheese Omelette (without sides)	460	33	2	9	680
DUNKIN' DONUTS					
Multigrain Bagel	390	8	9	65	560
Egg White Veggie Flatbread	280	10	3	32	690
Egg White Turkey Sausage Flatbread	280	8	3	32	770
EINSTEIN BROS.					
Power Bagel (plain)	310	5	4	61	280
Potato Salad	160	12	1	13	360
Good Grains Bagel (plain)	280	2.5	3	58	440
Pumpernickel Bagel (plain)	240	1.5	3	53	490
JAMBA JUICE					
Fresh Banana Oatmeal	280	4	6	57	20
Plain Oatmeal with Brown Sugar	220	3.5	5	44	20
Blueberry & Blackberry Oatmeal	290	1	6	58	30
Coldbuster (16 oz)	240	1.5	3	56	20
Apple Cinnamon Oatmeal	290	4	5	60	25
Berry Topper (12 oz)	300	4.5	7	59	85
Mango Peach Topper (12 oz)	320	4.5	6	64	85
Protein Berry Workout (16 oz)	280	0	3	52	115
Chimichurri Chicken Wrap (without sauce)	410	9	2	66	710
Greens and Grain Wrap (without dressing)	580	12	9	99	630

	CALORIES	FAT	FIBER	CARBS	SODIUM
KFC					
Corn on the Cob (3")	70	0.5	2	16	0
Grilled Chicken (whole wing)	80	5	0	1	250
Green Beans	20	0	1	3	290
Grilled Chicken (breast)	210	8	0	0	460
Potato Salad	210	11	3	26	560
BBQ Baked Beans	210	1.5	8	41	780
McDONALD'S					
Snack Size Fruit & Walnut Salad	210	8	2	31	60
Fruit & Maple Oatmeal (without brown sugar)	260	4.5	5	48	115
NINETY NINE					
Side of Broccoli Florets	30	1	3	4	80
Side of Fresh Grilled Asparagus	30	0.5	2	3	230
Sweet Potato Fries (½ serving)	275	18	4	25	270
Side of Perfect Green Beans	70	4.5	3	6	310
Fit for You Herb Salmon & Vegetables	440	28	4	10	320
Minestrone Soup, cup (8 oz)	180	4.5	5	29	470
Small Plate Red Pepper Hummus Platter	280	10	10	38	500
Minestrone Soup, crock (12 oz)	240	5	7	38	670
Side of Rosemary Parmesan Fries (½ serving)	260	17.5	2.5	24.5	675
Baked Potato Without Toppings	230	4	6	50	750
Fit for You Mushroom Bleu Top Sirloin	490	33	5	10	750
Baked Potato with Sour Cream	290	9	6	51	770
NOODLES & COMPANY					
Penne Rosa Mediterranean Bowl (small)	420	13	8	60	550
Spaghetti American Bowl (small)	340	9	5	51	590
OLIVE GARDEN					
Linguine alla Marinara (lunch portion)	310	4	5	55	670
Pasta e Fagioli	130	2.5	6	17	680
ORANGE JULIUS					
Bananarilla (16 oz)	320	7	5	65	70
Berry-Pom Twilight (20 oz)	230	0	5	55	70
Berry Banana Squeeze (20 oz)	270	0	4	70	10

	CALORIES	FAT	FIBER	CARBS	SODIUM
PANDA EXPRESS					
Steamed Rice with Mixed Veggies	490	0.5	5	106	530
Mixed Veggies	70	0.5	5	13	530
Eggplant Tofu Entree	310	24	3	19	680
Thai Cashew Chicken Breast Entree	240	12	2	14	640
Broccoli Chicken Entree	180	9	3	11	670
Broccoli Beef Entree	130	4	3	13	740
Sweet and Sour Pork Entree	450	26	3	40	400
PANERA					
Strawberry Granola Parfait	310	11	3	44	100
Grilled Egg & Cheese Sandwich	380	14	2	43	620
Creamy Tomato Soup with Croutons	370	12	5	39	740
Asian Sesame Chicken Salad	400	20	3	31	810
Breakfast Power Sandwich	330	14	4	31	830
Fuji Apple Chicken Salad	520	31	5	36	830
Grilled Chicken Caesar Salad (without dressing)	360	14	3	27	640
Dressing	150	2.5	0	2	190
PF CHANG'S					
Buddha's Feast Steamed with Brown Rice (½ order of lunch bowl)	210	2	5	39	80
Spicy Green Beans (small)	110	6	4	13	720
QUIZNO'S					
Cantina Chicken Sammie	285	5	2	27	490
Veggie Sammie	330	19	3	29	755
Raspberry Vinaigrette Chicken Chopped Salad (small)	330	12	2	37	760
Chili (cup)	185	4.5	3	23	770
Chicken Bacon Ranch Sammie	380	19	1	28	780
Honey Bourbon Chicken Sub (small)	300	5	2	45	790
RUBY TUESDAY'S					
Plain Grilled Chicken	240	4	0	0	75
Baked Potato (plain)	282	2	10	46	113
Plain Grilled Salmon	245	11	1	0	129

	CALORIES	FAT	FIBER	CARBS	SODIUM
Sugar Snap Peas	113	6	3	6	202
Fresh Steamed Broccoli	91	6	3	5	227
White Cheddar Mashed Potatoes	169	10	2	19	520
Creamy Mashed Cauliflower	136	8	3	10	714
Petite Grilled Salmon Salad	322	14	6	20	794
STARBUCKS					
Starbucks Perfect Oatmeal (without toppings)	140	2.5	4	25	105
Strawberry & Blueberry Yogurt Parfait	300	3.5	3	60	130
Protein Artisan Snack Plate	370	19	4	36	470
Chicken and Hummus Snack Plate	250	9	5	27	520
Apple Bran Muffin	350	9	7	64	520
Reduced-Fat Turkey Bacon with Egg Whites on English Muffin	320	7	3	43	700
Roasted Vegetable Panini	350	12	4	48	770
SUBWAY					
6" Oven Roasted Chicken Sandwich	320	4.5	5	49	750
Veggie Delite Mini Sub	150	1.5	3	30	280
Egg White & Cheese Muffin Melt	140	3.5	5	18	490
6" Veggie Delite with Swiss	280	7	5	45	440
6" Veggie Delite	230	2.5	5	45	410
TACO BELL					
Fresco Crunchy Taco	150	7	3	13	350
Fresco Soft Taco	190	7	4	22	580
Fresco Chicken Soft Taco	170	4	3	22	680
UNO CHICAGO GRILL					
Farro Salad (1 serving)	90	6	1	8	310
Roasted Eggplant, Spinach & Feta Thin Crust Pizza on Five-Grain Crust (⅓ of pizza)	290	11	4	38	560
Chopped Power Salad (½ order)	270	7	5	32	610
Roasted Vegetable & Feta Wrap (⅔ of wrap)	290	15	9	32	820

	CALORIES	FAT	FIBER	CARBS	SODIUM
WENDY'S					
Apple Pecan Chicken Salad (½ serving)	340	18	4	28	830
Broccoli and Cheese Potato	330	2	8	69	470
Sour Cream and Chives Potato	320	4	7	63	50
Grilled Chicken Go Wrap	260	10	1	25	750
Garden Side Salad with Italian Vinaigrette, Light Classic Ranch, Fat Free French, or Pomegranate Vinaigrette (without croutons)					
Salad:	25	0	2	5	30
Dressings:	31	0–6	0	4–9	200

The CarbLovers Quick & Easy Workout

YES, YOU WILL LOSE WEIGHT ON *THE CarbLovers Diet* without pumping iron or running a marathon. But you'll drop pounds faster if you exercise. The good news is that a diet rich in carbs fuels your muscles and gives you a natural energy boost, so you'll feel like leading a healthier, more active life. Here's a super-simple plan to keep you in shape.

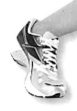

Monday/Wednesday/Friday/Saturday

Do one of the following cardio activities, in the intervals suggested, for maximum fat and calorie burn:

■ Alternate 2 minutes of brisk walking with 2 minutes of running for a total of 24 minutes.

■ On your bike, alternate 2 minutes of cycling at a moderate pace with 2 minutes of cycling at a fast pace for a total of 20 minutes.

■ On the elliptical trainer, alternate 2 minutes at moderate intensity with 2 minutes at vigorous intensity for a total of 24 minutes.

Tuesday/Thursday

Do this 15-minute, full-body strength routine—so simple it requires no equipment! Do 1 set of each exercise, resting for 30 to 60 seconds between exercises.

■ **PUSH-UP:** Lie on your stomach with your hands just outside your shoulders, elbows bent to 45 degrees, and fingers spread. Your toes should be tucked under, with your legs straight and abs pulled in. (For less of a challenge, start on your hands and knees.) Take a deep breath and push yourself up, keeping your body in a straight line (don't jut your butt up or let your belly sag). Slowly lower yourself down to starting position. Do 12 to 15 reps.

■ **CURTSY LUNGE:** Stand with your feet hip-width apart and hands on hips. Step diagonally back with your left foot and cross it behind your right; bend your knees (as if curtsying) as you reach your left hand to the outside of your right foot. Return to start. Do 15 reps, switch sides, and repeat.

■ **SIDE PLANK:** Lie on your right side with your legs stacked on top of one another and your right arm bent, with the elbow directly underneath the right shoulder for support and the forearm on the floor. Keeping your body completely aligned, draw your abs in and lift your hips to raise your body off the floor. Hold this position for 10 to 15 seconds, then lower back down to the floor and repeat on the other side; that's one rep. Do 2 to 3 reps.

■ **SQUAT:** Stand with your feet hip-width apart and your hands on your hips. Bend your knees and lower your butt down and back, as if sitting in a chair. Stop when your thighs are parallel to the floor (keep your knees behind your toes), pause, then rise back up. Do 15 to 20 reps.

■ **BICYCLE CRUNCH:** Lie on your back with your knees bent, feet on the floor, and hands behind your head (don't clasp your fingers). Press your lower back into the floor and tighten your abs as you lift your head, shoulders, and upper back off the floor and simultaneously move your right elbow and left knee toward each other while straightening the right leg (keep it off the ground). Draw your right knee back up and move your left elbow and right knee toward each other while straightening your left leg; that's one rep. Do 20 to 30 reps.

Sunday: Rest!

NOTE: Please get clearance from your doctor before starting The CarbLovers Quick & Easy Workout, especially if you have been inactive for a while.

CarbLovers for Life!

CONGRATULATIONS! YOU'VE REACHED YOUR GOAL WEIGHT, and you look and feel amazing. But you're probably already worrying about putting those pounds back on. Relax. We designed *CarbLovers* so that keeping those pounds off is super-easy. Think about it: On *CarbLovers,* you didn't cut out anything to slim down. Nothing was off-limits, so there aren't any foods to add back in—and no risk of a binge.

Maybe in the past you made the mistake of eating more or changing things up once you met your weight-loss goal. This time, you shouldn't feel that need. In Phase 2 of *The CarbLovers Diet* (The Immersion Plan), you consumed 1,600 calories a day and your daily target of Resistant Starch. To maintain your new, slender self, keep to those numbers.

> **CarbLovers Tip**
> Use the power of the Post-it to keep Resistant Starch in mind. Put notes on your fridge, mirror, dashboard, and wallet with messages like "Beans Are Beautiful" and "Bananas = Bikini Body."

Remember: You need less food to maintain your weight as your body gets lighter. So you can't go back to eating what it took to maintain, say, 160 pounds now that you weigh 130.

> **CarbLovers Tip**
> If your pants start feeling snug again, or you simply need some friendly support, go to carblovers.com for quick and easy weight-loss advice.

At the same time, now that you understand the *CarbLovers* philosophy, it's time to expand your horizons. Armed with a few simple rules, you can start creating your own meal plans and making smart food choices in restaurants, at your book club, on vacation, even at that tempting holiday party.

YOUR PERFECT CARBLOVERS MEAL

Make at Least One Perfect Meal Every Day!

To maintain your goal weight, it's important to consume these four key ingredients daily, at one sitting. They will work together to keep you slim! But please pay attention to portion size—you'll find the right portions for each of these superfoods in the chart on pages 144–45.

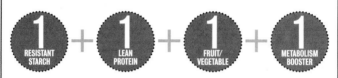

1 RESISTANT STARCH + **1** LEAN PROTEIN + **1** FRUIT/VEGETABLE + **1** METABOLISM BOOSTER

Three More Things to Keep in Mind

1. When choosing among grains and starches, always choose Resistant Starch (see charts, pages 146 and 150) or high-fiber carbs (see chart, page 147) over highly refined starches such as regular pasta (made from refined flour), white rice, white bread, and low-fiber breakfast cereals.

2. Choose high-performance fats such as monounsaturated fatty acids (MUFAs) and omega-3 fatty acids (see lists, pages 148–49). You've been hearing about them (and, we hope, eating them) for years: the "good fat" foods such as avocados, olives and olive oil, fatty fish (e.g., anchovies and salmon), peanuts, seeds and nuts, and coconut products. Use olive oil on salads instead of other oils; substitute guacamole or hummus for butter and mayo as a sandwich spread.

3. To add flavor to various dishes, go for metabolism boosters like peanut butter, coconut milk, cayenne pepper, vinegar, or anchovy paste.

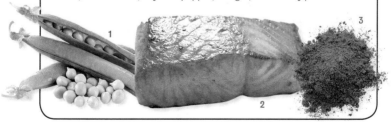

CarbLovers Portion Sizes (At a Glance)

Make sure to include one from each of these four groups in one meal every day. It's important to eat them at one sitting.

HIGH RESISTANT STARCH CHOICES
(150 calories)
Banana, slightly green, 1 large
Barley, ¾ cup
Beans, ½ cup
Bread, whole grain, 2 slices
(1-oz slices)
English muffin, whole wheat, 1
Tortilla chips, corn, 1 oz
Cornflakes, 1¼ cups
Puffed wheat, 2½ cups
Polenta, ⅔ cup cooked
Crispbread crackers, 4
Lentils, ½ cup cooked
Millet, ¾ cup cooked
Brown rice, ¾ cup cooked
Oatmeal, ½ cup uncooked
(1 cup cooked)
Pasta, whole wheat, 1 cup cooked
Peas, 1 cup cooked
Plantain, ¾ cup
Popcorn, 3 cups popped
Potato chips, 1 oz
Potato, 1 small baked
Potatoes, 1 cup cooked and cooled
Tortillas, 2 corn (6")
Yams, 1 cup cubed and cooked

LEAN PROTEIN CHOICES
(cooked, 150 calories)
Poultry, 3 oz skinless
Fish (especially salmon), 3 oz
Beef, 2 oz lean
Edamame, ½ cup
Tofu, ¾ cup
Soy crumbles, 1 cup
Eggs, 2

METABOLISM-BOOSTING CHOICES
(100 calories or less)
Avocado, ⅓ cup
Olive oil, 1 TBSP
Nuts or seeds, ⅛ cup
Peanut butter, 1 TBSP
Almond butter, 1 TBSP
Coconut milk, 3 TBSP
Shredded coconut, ⅓ cup
Chocolate, ¼ bar
Flaxseeds or ground flaxseeds,
2 TBSP
Low-fat yogurt, ¾ cup
Low-fat cheese, 1 slice
Low-fat milk, 1 cup
Low-fat soft cheese
(ricotta, cottage, etc), ½ cup
Whole fruit, 1 small
Sliced fruit, 1 cup
Dried fruit, ½ cup

PRODUCE CHOICES

Vegetables
(unlimited portion sizes)

Artichokes
Asparagus
Bean sprouts
Bok choy
Broccoli
Brussels sprouts
Cabbage
Carrots
Cauliflower
Celery
Collard greens
Cucumbers
Dark green leafy lettuce
Eggplant
Green or red bell peppers
Iceberg lettuce
Kale
Mesclun
Mushrooms
Mustard greens
Okra
Onions
Romaine lettuce
Spinach
Tomatoes
Turnip greens
Watercress
Wax beans
Zucchini

Fruit
Any medium whole fruit
Berries or sliced fruit, 1 cup

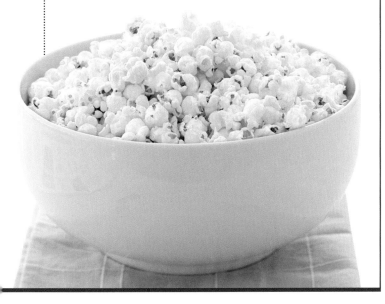

Top Resistant Starch Foods

FOOD	CALORIES	SERVING SIZE	GRAMS RS
Banana, slightly green	105	1 medium (7–8")	12.5g
Banana, ripe	105	1 medium (7–8")	4.7g
Oatmeal, uncooked/toasted	153	½ cup	4.6g
Beans, white, cooked/canned	124	½ cup	3.8g
Lentils, cooked	115	½ cup	3.4g
Potatoes, cooked and cooled	118	1 potato, 2.5" diameter	3.2g
Plantain, cooked	89	½ cup, slices	2.7g
Beans, garbanzo, cooked/canned	143	½ cup	2.1g
Pasta, whole wheat, cooked	174	1 cup	2.0g
Barley, pearled, cooked	97	½ cup	1.9g
Pasta, white, cooked and cooled	221	1 cup	1.9g
Beans, kidney, cooked/canned	112	½ cup	1.8g
Potatoes, boiled with skin	118	1 potato, 2.5" diameter	1.8g
Rice, brown, cooked	109	½ cup	1.7g
Beans, pinto, cooked/canned	122	½ cup	1.6g
Peas, canned/frozen	62	½ cup	1.6g
Pasta, white, cooked	221	1 cup	1.5g
Beans, black, cooked/canned	114	½ cup	1.5g
Millet, cooked	104	½ cup	1.5g
Potatoes, baked (skin and flesh)	130	1 small	1.4g
Bread, pumpernickel	71	1-oz slice	1.3g
Corn polenta, cooked	113	½ cup	1.0g
Peas, black-eyed, cooked	80	½ cup	1.0g
Potato chips	158	1 oz	1.0g
Quinoa, cooked	111	½ cup	1.0g
Yam, cooked	79	½ cup cubes	1.0g
Cornflakes	100	1 cup	0.9g
Bread, rye (whole)	73	1-oz slice	0.9g
Puffed wheat	55	1¼ cup	0.9g
Crackers, rye crispbread	101	½ cup crushed	0.8g
Tortillas, corn	62	1 oz, 6" tortilla	0.8g
English muffin	134	1 whole muffin	0.7g
Bread, sourdough	82	1-oz slice	0.6g
Crackers, rye crispbread	73	2 crispbreads	0.6g
Oatmeal, cooked	166	1 cup	0.5g
Couscous, cooked and chilled	88	½ cup	0.4g
Bread, whole grain	75	1-oz slice	0.3g

Top Fiber Foods

The following foods are all naturally rich in fiber. Both the calorie and fiber amounts are given per 1 cup

FOOD	CALORIES	GRAMS OF FIBER
Artichokes	76	14g
Avocado	276	12.9g
Barley, pearled, cooked	193	6g
Beans, baked, canned	368	10g
Beans, black, cooked	228	15g
Beans, great northern, cooked	209	12g
Beans, kidney, cooked	225	11g
Beans, pinto, cooked	244	15g
Beans, navy, cooked	255	19g
Beans, white, cooked	299	13g
Buckwheat flour, whole groat	402	12g
Bulgur, cooked	151	8g
Chickpeas (garbanzo beans), cooked	268	13g
Dates, chopped	415	12g
Figs, dried	371	14.6g
Lentils, cooked, boiled, without salt	230	16g
Lima beans, large, cooked	216	13g
Oat bran, raw	231	15g
Peas, split, cooked	231	16g
Raspberries, frozen	64	11g
Refried beans, canned, vegetarian	201	11g
Soup, beans with ham, canned, chunky, ready to serve	231	11g
Wheat flour, whole grain	407	15g

Top Monounsaturated Fatty Acid (MUFA) Foods

These foods are naturally rich in MUFA.

FOOD	CALORIES	SERVING SIZE	MUFA
Avocados	322	1 avocado	20g
Macadamia nuts, dry roasted	203	1 oz (10–12 nuts)	16.8g
Semisweet chocolate chips	806	1 cup	16.7g
Hazelnuts or filberts	178	1 oz (21 nuts)	12.9g
Pecans	196	1 oz (20 halves)	11.6g
Pork, spareribs	337	3 oz	11.5g
Pork, ribs	314	3 oz	11.4g
Lamb, chops	305	3 oz	10.6g
Olive oil	119	1 TBSP	9.9g
Ricotta cheese	428	1 cup	8.9g
Canola oil	124	1 TBSP	8.9g
Almonds	163	1 oz (23 nuts)	8.8g
Salmon	335	½ fillet	8.2g
Cashews	163	1 oz (18 nuts)	7.7g
Peanuts	166	1 oz (28 nuts)	7.4g
Brazil nuts	186	1 oz (6–8 nuts)	7.0g
Pistachios	162	1 oz (49 nuts)	6.9g
Sunflower seed kernels	186	¼ cup	3.0g

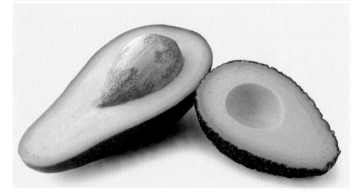

Top Omega-3 Fatty Acid Foods

These are the planet's richest foods in omega-3 fatty acids,
ranked from most to least.

FOOD	CALORIES	SERVING SIZE	OMEGA-3
Walnuts	185	1 oz	2.6g
Mackerel, canned, drained	177	4 oz	1.5g
Salmon	184	3 oz	1.2g
Tuna, canned	109	3 oz	0.7g
Fish, herring, Atlantic, kippered	62	1 oz	0.6g
Anchovies	60	1 oz	0.6g
Pollack	100	3 oz	0.5g
Flounder	99	3 oz	0.5g
Clams	126	3 oz	0.3g
Shrimp	84	3 oz	0.3g
Haddock	95	3 oz	0.2g
Catfish	89	3 oz	0.2g
Cod	89	3 oz	0.1g

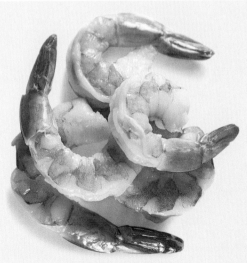

Score a Perfect RS 10

The meals in The *CarbLovers* Kickstart and Immersion Plans add up to at least 10 grams of Resistant Starch a day. But it's easy to get all the Resistant Starch you need on your own! Just use the list of high Resistant Starch carbs on page 146, along with the nutritional information with the *CarbLovers* recipes, to count Resistant Starch grams and make sure your menu adds up to a slimmer you. Here's a quick cheat sheet.

BREAKFAST CARBS	+	LUNCH CARBS	+	DINNER CARBS	=	10+ GRAMS OF RESISTANT STARCH PER DAY
1 banana (**4.7g**) in a smoothie		½ cup white beans (**3.8g**)		1 serving whole-wheat pasta (**2g**)		10.5g
1 banana (**4.7g**) with oatmeal (**0.5g**)		Sandwich on rye bread (**1.8g**)		½ cup brown rice (**1.7g**) + ½ cup black beans (**1.5g**)		10.2g
Cornflakes (**0.9g**) with banana (**4.7g**)		Ham, Pear & Swiss Cheese Sandwich (**2.6g**)		½ cup barley (**1.9g**)		10.1g
Banana & Almond Butter Toast (**5.6g**)		Black Bean & Zucchini Quesadillas (**4.7g**)		Baked potato (**1.4g**)		11.7g
Granola with Pecan, Pumpkinseeds & Dried Mango (**5g**)		Three-Bean Soup with Canadian Bacon (**4g**)		Pasta with Peas, Ham & Parmesan Cheese (**4g**)		13g
Banana-Nut Oatmeal + 1 slice rye bread, toasted (**6.1g**)		Sandwich on pumpernickel bread (**2g**) + 1 oz potato chips (**1g**)		½ cup millet (**1.5g**)		10.6g
Blueberry Oat Pancakes with Maple Yogurt (**4.6g**)		Banana-Nut Elvis Wrap (**3g**)		Black Bean Tacos (**4.7g**)		12.3g

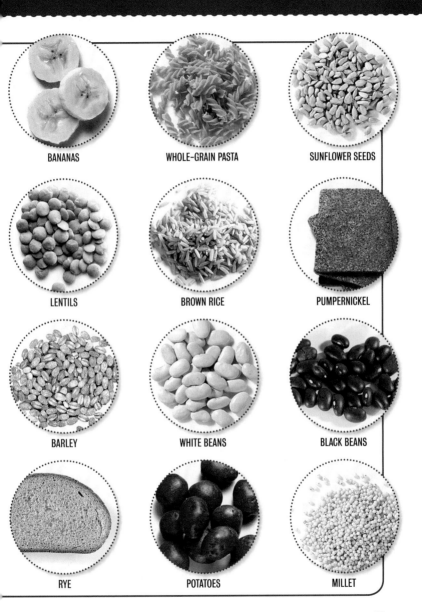

BANANAS

WHOLE-GRAIN PASTA

SUNFLOWER SEEDS

LENTILS

BROWN RICE

PUMPERNICKEL

BARLEY

WHITE BEANS

BLACK BEANS

RYE

POTATOES

MILLET

"I Lost Weight On CarbLovers"

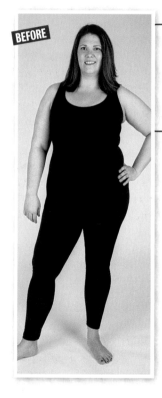

BEFORE

MICHELLE FERRELL
Age: 33
Height: 5'10"
Weight before: 240
Weight after: 190
Pounds lost: 50

Biggest success moment: Buying boots! My legs had never been small enough to wear the styles I liked. I paired the boots with a new dress for Thanksgiving dinner, and everyone kept telling me how great I looked. It felt so good to hear that my hard work had paid off.

Biggest challenge: Learning how to eat in a way that's healthy and gluten-free. While a lot of *The CarbLovers Diet* includes wheat and rye (things I can't eat), making substitutions is easier than I expected.

Favorite recipes: I love the Shrimp Stir-Fry with Ginger (page 88), so I make it using gluten-free La Choy Lite Soy Sauce. For the Chicken Pita Sandwich (page 69), I substitute a Food for Life Brown Rice Tortilla for the whole-grain pita.

My weight has always been up and down. I would lose 30 pounds by not eating very much, then gain it all back once I started eating regularly again. *CarbLovers* worked because it was a lifestyle change.

Learning how to cook was the key to my success. Before, I would just eat whatever was convenient—big bowls of cereal, fast food, or anything I could pop in the microwave. I never knew it was so easy to cook a healthy meal. My boyfriend has been trying to eat healthier, and he loves the *Carb-Lovers* recipes, too.

AFTER

Following the recipes means I don't have to count calories. And since the meals taste so good, it doesn't seem like a diet. Instead of feeling deprived, I feel like I'm embarking on this new, healthy-eating lifestyle.

I've always been scared that even if I lost weight, I might fall off the wagon and gain it all back. But I've learned that even if I do make a mistake, I can just start over the next day.

When I started the diet, I wore a size 20. After a couple weeks, none of my clothes fit. I had to clean out my closet and start anew—that was a huge moment for me. I wear a size 16 now. In the past, I would hang on to my bigger clothes because my weight fluctuated so much, but this time I'm going to give them all away. It gives me a reason to keep going—I don't want to be in those clothes again!

Subject Index

154

Acknowledgments

THE SUCCESS OF *THE CARBLOVERS DIET* CONFIRMED WHAT I ALREADY KNEW: that achieving and maintaining a healthy weight without hunger is something that *Health* magazine's and Health.com's 20 million readers truly care about. *CarbLovers Diet* fans told me they wanted more—more recipes, new diet plans, and lots of restaurant, entertaining, and grab-and-go eating options. So here it all is! We started researching *The CarbLovers Diet Pocket Guide* just a few months after the original book went to press, and we've continued to update it until the last possible moment because we want this to be a diet you can stick with—and enjoy—wherever you are and wherever you go!

Of course, many people helped create this incredible weight-loss resource. Thanks goes to *Health*'s food and nutrition editor and my coauthor, Frances Largeman-Roth, RD, and our team of nutrition and culinary experts: Sonthe Burge, RD, Adeena Sussman, and Abby Gerstein, RD. Also a big thanks to Susan Toepfer, who was instrumental in updating and adding important new recipes and advice to *CarbLovers*. Thanks to Kate Stinchfield for her invaluable research. A shout-out goes to the *Health* staff, who worked on *The CarbLovers Diet Pocket Guide* while putting out a great magazine: Ben Margherita, Marc Einsele, Marybeth Dulany, Sung Choi, Su Reid-St. John, Sarah DiGiulio, Leslie Barrie, as well as Amy O'Connor, editor in chief of Health.com, and copy editor Jim Cholakis. We also want to thank Sylvia Auton and John L. Brown for being such wonderful supporters of *Health* and giving us the tools we needed to create this book. Thanks, too, to the terrific teams at Time Home Entertainment Inc. and Oxmoor House: Richard Fraiman, Jim Childs, Tom Mifsud, Steven Sandonato, Susan Payne Dobbs, Fonda Hitchcock, Holly Smith, and Laurie Herr.

Frances wants to give a thank-you to Rhonda Witwer at National Starch Food Innovation and to Hope Warshaw, RD, for sharing their Resistant Starch knowledge. Finally, our deepest gratitude goes to those who lost big on *The CarbLovers Diet* and helped us fine-tune it so that millions could experience the thrill of getting slim while eating carbs. We couldn't have done it without you!

Ellen Kunes
Editor in Chief, *Health* magazine
Editorial Director, Health.com

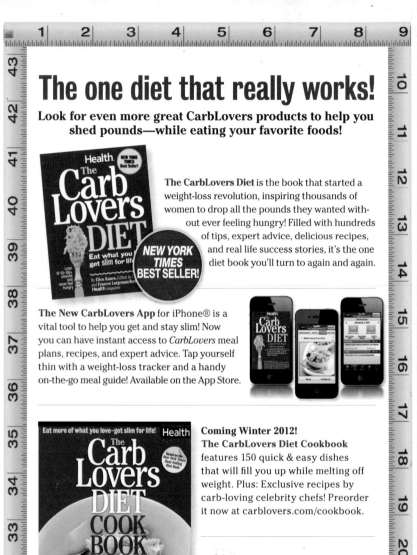